Biohack Your Mood with Plant-Based Food
*Optimize Your Mental Health with Targeted
Nutrition and Gut Support*

by Joshua Flowers

healthymoods.org

ISBN: 979-8-9895573-1-8 (paperback)
ISBN: 979-8-9895573-0-1 (ePub)

Connect

No matter what stage you're in with your food-mood journey, I would love to have you join the Healthy Moods community! Mental health issues are not something to be ashamed of. At Healthy Moods, we believe that it's important to have a safe and open community to share the successes and challenges that are part of working through mental health concerns and implementing change.

We also know that there can be lots of shame around food and dieting. It can be hard to talk about goals we have struggled to achieve for many years. People can be opinionated about what diet works best. We want to encourage an open dialogue no matter what your dietary preferences are or how many attempts you've had at making the changes you would like for your life. We're here to offer support along the way.

So come find us on Instagram @healthy.moods and Facebook @healthymoods and let us know what questions you have or what information you would like to share. If you prefer a 1:1 approach, you can schedule individual therapy sessions at healthymoods.org as well.

Be sure to sign up for our newsletter to receive our getting started guide, which includes additional recipes and tips. This way, you won't miss out on updates including free giveaways of our Plant-Based Programs for Anxiety, as well as stays at our Veg Retreat and Rentals in Portugal!

Sign up at healthymoods.org/free-ebook

Finally, we are super excited to share our chatbot, the Food Mood Guru, with you! He makes a great companion on this food-mood journey. Check out healthymoods.org/food-mood-chatbot to ask him any questions you may have!

Contents

Getting Started

The Choice

Would you rather eat your vegetables or someone else's poo? Guessing that isn't a hard one to answer. Though if you chose the latter, no judgment here. But, if poo is not for you, and you are not eating your veggies—or the amount you need to get the necessary nutrients and fiber that the trillions of hungry microorganisms in your gut are starving for—then you may not have much choice in the matter.

We'll get to the specifics of why this is a decision you may be faced with in the future, but for now, let's devise a game plan so you can avoid eating poo should you feel that is the best option for your life.

It all starts with something we have a choice about each and every day: what we put into our mouth or, more importantly, our gut. The options seem limitless, at least if we were born into a life where food is so abundant that we don't have to think about where the next meal will come from. Many of us have become so accustomed to having unlimited access to food that we don't stop to consider if that food is helping us feel our best.

For those who already eat healthily, it is still easy to get overwhelmed by conflicting diet information and ever-changing health fads. And while there is good science out there about how to eat to lose weight, build muscle, or avoid a heart attack, the science on the connection between diet and mental health is limited.

The good news is that we are entering an era where we are more and more aware of the link between food and mood. The emerging field of nutritional psychology is providing us with new data that we can use to understand how food impacts our mental well-being. Even if you already eat a healthy diet, the studies can help you further hone your food choices to address specific mental health concerns that may benefit from targeted nutrition. These are exciting times to explore our relationship with food, ourselves, and the microbial world we depend on.

We'll begin our exploration by looking at some factors contributing to the social, environmental, and personal breakdowns that have led to the current health crisis. As we consider a response, we'll do this through a lens of hope while embracing a mindful and compassionate stance.

In Chapter 2, I'll walk you through a brief overview of the systems involved in this food-mood dance. You'll be introduced to the many players waiting to work with you in a symbiotic orchestra of health and wellness. It's a classic example of "scratch my back, I'll scratch yours." When we eat foods that our gut bugs love, they return the favor by initiating a cascade of molecular interactions that are instrumental in cleaning and repairing, supporting our immune system, and even lifting us up mentally and emotionally.

We've got a finite amount of time on this spinning planet—which seems to be picking up its rotational speed at an unprecedented clip. Since you're reading this book, I'm guessing you want to be mindful of how you use your time here while applying a few healthy changes along the way. In Chapter 3, we'll dive deeper into strategies for change and consider various ways to make the process enjoyable, further building on concepts introduced later in this chapter.

By Chapter 4, you'll be well-equipped with enough knowledge to start taking action. I'll give you some tips and tricks to help you optimize your mental and emotional health with plant-based food. For the past four years, I have been reading anything I can about the subject and applying different strategies to my diet. I want to use what I've learned to help you cut right to the chase, so you can start making changes that allow you to feel better now.

It can often feel like we are getting squeezed tight, trying to keep up with everything life throws our way —especially if we experience the challenges of depression, anxiety, and mental fatigue. This becomes even more difficult when we also struggle to get enough sleep. What can be a real kick in the genitals is when all these things show up while you are trying to blow off a bit of steam in the bedroom—and the parts of you that need to be on board with the idea aren't.

In Chapter 5, we'll focus on using plant-based food to target symptoms of anxiety, depression, mental fatigue, insomnia, and low libido. You'll learn which micronutrients are best for addressing these mental health issues and which foods are rich sources of them. Then, we'll combine some of these foods to create a few recipes and daily menus. The recipes will be simple and stress-free, using fewer than ten main ingredients and taking less than half an hour to make.

If, by that point, you feel inspired and wish to go further, Chapter 6 will provide ideas beyond diet choices that can help support your gut and the planet's health.

So, while the world spins madly on, we're going to try to slow down a little and see if we can make sense of what is most important here: find out what this food-mood dance is all about; try to get at a simple, working understanding of this complicated process; and start exploring eating-strategies to optimize your mental and emotional wellness.

But first, we need to start with what we are up against.

The Poo Pill

Because the human species has not been the best stewards of this wonderful world we've been plopped down upon, other species are disappearing at a rapid rate. As of this writing, 27% of all mammals[1] and 30% of tree species[2] are holding on for dear life. Scientists are concerned that our monoculture-obsessed agricultural system may also have us on track to lose valuable plant species. In response, they've built a seed warehouse. Think of it as Noah's Ark for seeds. If we continue the course we're on and erase certain plants as we did the ivory-billed woodpecker, these scientists are making sure we can resurrect certain plant foods—should we decide that they were an integral part of this symbiotic system after all.

The same thing happening in the natural world is happening to our bodies: bacterial species are being wiped out. We became obsessed with cleanliness—got a little OCD with it. Just as we made the environment less wild by fencing out or killing off everything we deemed a threat, we tried to tame our microbiome, a vast community of microorganisms that had made our bodies their home.

---

[1] https://www.iucnredlist.org/
[2] https://www.bgci.org/news-events/bgci-launches-the-state-of-the-worlds-trees-report/

True, some of the species were an actual threat. But, like we tend to do, we went overboard with the domination and subjugation thing. Antibiotics, soap, and sterilization techniques have their place. But we were arrogant, disregarded the wisdom of our bodies —which naturally gravitate toward homeostasis—and set out on a perpetual warpath. In so doing, we created an imbalance by also wiping out some of the soldiers that had been on our side: millions of little gut-troopers monitoring invasions, manufacturing their arsenal of chemical concoctions, and engaging in the battle for a peaceful state within our bodies.

While we exterminated some of the critters in our gut, our agricultural system was helping to starve the poor things by depleting the nutrients they relied on for food. This resulted from the same backward logic that progress involves eradicating crucial team members. This team was also made up of a complex system of microorganisms living in the layers of our soil. Just as we disregarded the wisdom of our bodies, the wisdom of the earth—which seeks abundance for all organisms —was also not consulted. Misguided farming practices plundered the masterfully crafted systems thriving in the topsoil.

The widespread practices of monocropping, coupled with the intensive use of pesticides and herbicides, have compromised the health of the soil microbiome. This situation parallels the delicate balance in our gut: both ecosystems need specific elements for healthy functioning. When these elements are depleted or missing, these systems can become unbalanced, leading to a state known as dysbiosis—an imbalance between beneficial and harmful microorganisms. This puts the immediate environment at risk and threatens the broader interconnected systems.

The miracle of the soil results from nature's ability to give and take in a way that allows the whole system to flourish. Through nutrient cycling, plants extract but also replace specific minerals. This dynamic relationship with the soil allows plants to create the nutrients we absorb when consuming them.

The soil's diversity benefits from rotating crops on a particular plot of land. This is because the same plant isn't sucking up the same nutrients year after year. When this doesn't happen, as with monocropping, the soil becomes depleted of certain minerals. And why does this matter? This type of soil leads to plants that are less diverse in their nutrient makeup.

A diverse soil microbiome is vital for nutrient-rich crops. So too, a diverse gut microbiome is essential for our health. Our gut's microbiota (bacteria, viruses, protozoa, and fungi) need various nutrients to work their magic. But what they are getting due to the poor quality soil, resulting in less nutrient-dense plants, are less than optimal meals. All the microorganisms that constitute the microbiome in our gut have specific tasks that keep our systems well-tuned. This includes everything from how we digest and absorb nutrients to how we heal and feel. What we feed them will determine how well these jobs get done.

Pouring loads of antibiotics down our throats and

following the Standard American Diet (SAD)—which includes too many "foods" with all the helpful nutrients processed right out of them—has led to the concern that we have lost much of the microbial diversity needed to help us stay healthy and happy.

Recognizing this issue, scientists have established the Microbiota Vault, akin to the seed vault that preserves plant diversity for future generations. The Microbiota Vault warehouses little air-tight containers of fecal matter—teeming with rare microorganisms—hanging out in a carefully controlled environment. The goal is to preserve these microbial "treasures" for a future where we may need to reinvigorate our depleted gut microbiomes. And how will this be accomplished? Fecal microbiota transplants (FMTs), or poo-pills, if you will.

FMTs are a novel medical intervention in which fecal matter, rich with beneficial gut bacteria, is transferred from a healthy donor into a recipient. This transfer takes place via capsules or enemas. The goal is to replenish the recipient's gut with a diverse microbiome to improve various health conditions.

The concept of FMTs is brilliant (certainly puts a unique twist on the zero-waste idea), but it doesn't have to be our only option. We can nurture a healthy gut microbiome by making mindful food choices. In doing so, you could be sitting on a potential goldmine: a healthy and diverse gut microbiome could make you a valuable donor—next side hustle, perhaps?

Joking aside, these systems are resilient and are

worth more than gold. We should treat them as such.

There's Hope

Fortunately, nature is designed so that biological systems can adapt and respond to change. In the same way our brains can forge new neural connections when we stop exposing them to harmful substances, the soil can rejuvenate its nutrients through practices like crop rotation and mineral replenishment. Similarly, our gut microbiome recalibrates when we reduce our intake of processed foods and increase our consumption of nutrient-rich foods packed with fiber, prebiotics, and beneficial bacteria.

Though science continues to explore the nuanced relationship between diet and mood, we are only beginning to understand the intricate process where gut bacteria metabolize micronutrients and prebiotics to produce neurochemicals. However, you and I don't need to know which specific bacterial strains produce which neurochemicals. Instead, we will focus on creating a relationship with our food that nourishes our system rather than depletes it. This way, we can build protections against feeling sick, sad, anxious, and tired.

By becoming more conscious of where our food comes from and choosing types of food that provide quality ingredients, we can improve our health and well-being. The foods we'll be focused on are plants.

As science advances, we're beginning to understand plant-based foods' complex genetic makeup and their unique phytonutrients. But again, we don't need to know about all the different types of nutrients (though we'll review some of the key ones for mental health). By broadening the variety of plants we eat, we increase the amount of these health-promoting compounds our bodies rely on.

Edible plants are crucial not only because they're unprocessed, low in sugar, and low in fat. They're also packed with anti-inflammatory properties, aid in toxin removal, are nutrient-dense, and are full of fiber— offering a feast for your microbes and a boost to your mental health.

The good news is that we can experience the benefits of dietary changes within days. This is why diet can be an excellent starting point for those seeking to feel better. Plus, it's foundational. Adding exercise or meditation can have tremendous benefits, but unlike eating, these activities aren't essential for survival. Eating three times a day gives you three opportunities to make choices that can impact how you feel.

So, there is hope. And plants can help. But it may be useful to know how we got here in the first place.

Arriving at This Point

As a mental health counselor, over the past 20 years, I have seen many people hurting. Unfortunately, there are no quick fixes. Many individuals work incredibly hard to feel a bit better. And the number of people facing similar challenges is increasing. Worldwide, over 10% of the population has a mental health disorder. The highest number, around 301 million people, are facing the overwhelm of anxiety, while another 280 million are weighed down by depression.[3]

There are many debates around the etiology of mental disorders, but the current theory suggests a biopsychosocial (and some add spiritual) influence. This is to say that *everything* contributes to the difficulties: it's a breakdown, on some level, in our biology, psychology, society, and spirituality. We are disconnected. And the result is a whole host of problems.

The process of disconnecting from important aspects of human experience goes back to the 4th century

---

[3] https://www.who.int/news-room/fact-sheets/detail/mental-disorders

when the church came up with the Sacrament of Penance. This was the bright idea that lay people had to go through the priests to communicate with God. In a sense, we eradicated God from daily life by removing people's direct relationship with the Divine and inserting an often misguided middleman. The layperson was discouraged from having an experience of the Divine. In fact, it was often a punishable offense. This was the first of many disconnections that cut us off from the relationships we depended on in more ways than we realized.

After severing the Divine connection, we set our sites on the land and the creatures that used it for their home. By the 18th century, the agricultural revolution was in full swing. We decided that taking control of a complex system by removing ourselves from it and then seeking to tame and dominate it was the best path forward. The church had no qualms, taking the stance that it was ours to have dominion over.

Once we secured our "rule" over the land and animals, we trained our sites on the body. The Victorians did a spectacular job of cultivating fear toward the multitude of wonders that our bodies possess. In so doing, they became quite removed from something they carried around with them every day. The church didn't help in this matter either. They placed the soul on a pedestal and pointed their long bony fingers at the innocent bystander: the flesh. The body became the culprit in many a-dirty-deed. With this view, we grew to judge and mistrust it. Disembodied in this fashion, we lost our ability to attune to its wisdom.

When told that "cleanliness was godliness," we didn't

bat an eye. We jumped in line to get our sanitization products, scrubbed down our homes and bodies with them, and took pills to rid our insides of any potential threat. We became obsessed with the desire to be safe from foreigners (in this case, bacteria).

Soon, we found ourselves disconnected from so many life-enhancing elements that the transition to embracing technology and the World Wide Web was ripe for complete entanglement. We were primed for wanting some form of connection, even if it wasn't exactly a direct line.

While in this tech trance, the Covid-19 pandemic hits, and we're instructed to isolate. And as shocking as the disconnection from one another was, we managed. We were being weaned off our need for one another (or at least, desensitized to the pain it was causing us). You would think this is about as bad as it gets. But is it?

Could our brains be next? Or even our words? Artificial Intelligence (AI) may create a gap between us and our human cognitive abilities. As we become increasingly reliant on superintelligent AI, we risk alienating ourselves from our minds. Furthermore, the ongoing 'war on words'—where cancel culture looms large—risks turning language into a feared entity, thereby distancing us from its creative and, indeed, occasionally offensive possibilities.

It has become a sad state of affairs, and our moods and nervous systems reflect just how sad.

How do we find our way back? How do we recapture

our relationship with these crucial elements of the human experience? The answer, or at least an essential first step, is food.

Food connects us. We start with the production, where we are in direct contact with the earth, soil, and all the natural elements that are transpiring to create the sugar, fats, and proteins that make up a particular food item, say, the humble potato. We (or the farmers) can change the game here by stepping back into the symbiotic dance and not only taking but giving back to the ecosystem. Through regenerative agriculture, practices like crop rotation, reducing tillage, composting, and cover cropping, can begin to rebalance depleted soil.

Eventually, the potato finds its way onto our plates as we engage in the time-honored tradition of "breaking bread," which is synonymous with communion. We may even pause for a moment to offer up a sense of gratitude (reconnecting with the Divine) before connecting with the food on our plate and the people who have joined us at the table.

And now, as that potato winds its way down through our intestinal tract, it will end up in our large intestine, the main hangout for the microbiota. As the potato is broken down, it offers up nutrients that will soon be traveling back into our system as little chemical messengers that will impact our emotional and mental state. Our gut also benefits from us sitting around the table with others, as we not only exchange words but bacteria that will help diversify our microbiome.

So, in this one act, we have established a bond with the earth, our bodies, one another, and, potentially, the Divine—having a biopsychosocial-spiritual impact on our well-being.

Sounds easy, right? Just eat more plants. Bonus if you do this with others. Yet, for many people, this is far from easy. I realized, even as someone who has been health-conscious for at least half my life, I rarely got enough fiber to appease the hungry critters in my colon.

Maybe it is better to say that the theory is simple— eating a wide range of plant-based foods to increase micro and macronutrients will, in turn, increase the microbial diversity in our microbiome, having an impact on our physical and mental health—but the practical application can be tricky.

I hope that by the time you finish reading this book, you will have concrete steps to make it easier. And that you will have some specific goals for sustainable habits that fit your unique genetic makeup and disposition.

Next, we'll consider a few principles as we begin this process of building habits that bring about change.

How We Change

The field of psychotherapy has gone through various phases where clinicians focused on a problem and then applied the treatment that was in vogue at the time. Most recently, they became enraptured with the brain. Thinking was identified as the problem, and cognitive behavioral therapy (CBT) was used to change the unhelpful thoughts. There's much to be in awe of when considering the brain and its cognitive processes. But we have given it god-like status over all the other impressive aspects of being human. And to a certain degree, this status seems to fit—it is "up there" running much of the show. But, the truth is it can't do it alone. And what we've realized in the last decade is that it definitely can't do it without two-way communication with our guts.

There are lots of things we can do to change. If we want to feel better, a whole world of wellness is waiting to sell us the solution. To a degree, I'm a part of that world. Though, I'll be the first to admit I don't have the solution. And, what works for me may not work for you. We are all unique, not only in how we think but also in how we experience our specific reality. This reality—that only you can know—can be your guide. Notice I said "reality." This is important because reality is not what you *think*, though we confuse the two all the time. What we think often separates us from reality because it is the experience (reality) getting filtered through judgments and perceptions. In other words, what we *think* about reality. And this thinking is a big part of the problem. In fact, it's what creates many of our problems in the first place (but that's a whole other book).

We give thinking too much credit and rely on it to inform us about how things are. But it's often wrong about how things are, and when we boil it down, we don't know much.

But our bodies do. They are a direct line to a more profound knowing. Call it intuition, a "gut" check, or an unconscious understanding. Whatever you call it, it is fundamental and can be an ally in self-discovery and transformation.

What I will be encouraging you to do in this whole process is think less. Less is more here. And by thinking less, I'm hoping you will get a sense of how your body speaks. It can often be quite subtle. It may even be speaking right now.

Try this: put this book down for a minute and tell yourself, "I'm going to try an experiment where I try thinking less and experiencing my reality more." As you say this, what do you feel? What are the sensations you notice in your body? Would you say it is more of openness or resistance? There is no wrong way to experience: either you feel open or closed, excited or fearful, light or heavy, etc. Some people have a hard time feeling anything at all. Even this is information. The point is to be curious and notice what comes up.

There is an innate skill called interoception, where we can direct our awareness to what's happening inside our bodies. It can take some practice, but we can all do it. Pause for a minute. Try to tune in to what the innermost part of your big toe feels like. Can you get a sense of its density? Does it feel heavy or light? Is it open or closed? If it had a personality, what do you imagine it would be? Maybe it has a memory of being stubbed one too many times and is a bit shy to step out into the world. Or does it feel resolute, ready to carry you into action? This is one example of how we can hone this skill by utilizing our creativity and curiosity.

Interoception can help as you read this book. Try to incorporate this way of experiencing: while you read, also notice how you feel inside; pay attention to what sensations come up. This can guide you. I could be feeding you a load of crap (and you may still be unsure about if you are down with consuming feces or not). If what I say doesn't resonate with your reality—if you notice yourself tense up, or even feel a surge of anger —listen to what that may be telling you.

This skill will be helpful when you start implementing some of the diet changes we'll discuss later. By tuning in to what your body "thinks" about the food you are ingesting, you will be accessing your body's wisdom, which is more important than any suggestion I make or any diet plan you believe you should follow.

As we step into the next part of this journey, let's try

to shift our focus from our overly analytical minds to our intuitive bodies. Our bodies hold a reservoir of wisdom that is often overlooked, a wisdom that can guide us toward better health decisions and a greater sense of well-being. It may feel unconventional, but consider this approach of less thinking and more feeling and sensing as an invitation to explore a different, perhaps more authentic, connection with yourself. The following section will examine an essential element of incorporating this approach into daily life.

Be Kind to You

Compassion. This will be the bedrock that we will build from. Always compassion. Force and ridicule create resistance and defeat. Be gentle with yourself. When you veer off course, kindly redirect yourself and realize you are not on the best path for your health and wellness.

We can cultivate compassion on many levels: how we think about ourselves and our situation, talk to ourselves, and stay in contact with ourselves by attuning to what is going on within. Start by being aware of your thoughts. Bonus points if you find yourself being a bit tyrannical and gently reverse course by trying a kinder approach.

Pausing and asking yourself, "How am I feeling now?" and paying attention to what you notice can be helpful. Eating mindfully by attuning to your food's textures and subtle flavors is a gift of compassion. We have ample opportunities to practice this way of being.

Less judgment and more observation are essential. It's hard to pay attention when too many things are happening. It is easy to get stuck in this cycle: we perceive that we suck in some way, feel we should be doing it better, and because we hold on to the lie that we are so far removed from where we should be, we pile on the tasks hoping that this will increase the speed in which we will achieve what we have deemed optimal. But trying to tackle many new habits simultaneously usually leads to a bunch of partial attempts. And none of the habits are sustained over the long term.

With habit formation, also, less is more. Start with one new behavior at a time. If the new behavior is a big jump from where you currently find yourself, break it down to a simple first step. If the SAD diet has been your go-to, start by adding one new plant-based food a week.

If you already feel that you have a healthy diet, try adding a day or two where you get more than the low recommendation of 25-35 grams of fiber. Shoot for a 38-50 grams a day.

When you are feeling confident with your healthy eating habits and increasing the diversity of plants you are consuming, you can get creative and experiment a bit: push your comfort level with a new recipe, include a new combination of foods that you didn't even know could work together; figure out what micronutrients you may be deficient in and use certain foods that are rich in them; see how many different colors you can include in a single meal.

Embracing this journey means experimenting, learning, and growing—taking small steps toward expanding your comfort zone over time. Be patient, be compassionate, and remember that every step, no matter how small, can bring you closer to your goals.

This process involves changes to your diet and a shift in your mindset and lifestyle, fostering a relationship with your body grounded in understanding, respect, and care.

In the coming chapters, we'll unlock surprising insights about how the foods we eat can transform our moods and overall well-being. You'll discover fascinating science, practical tips, and foods that can help you feel happier and healthier than ever before.

The Players

Neurotransmitters

We'll begin our exploration of the intricate relationship between mood and food with a dive into the world of neurobiology. This scientific field studies the nervous system's structure and function, shedding light on how it influences our behavior, emotions, and mental health.

The stars of this neurobiological show are the neurons, the specialized cells that send electrical signals from the brain to other body parts. Neurons are diligent messengers whose axons deliver signals, and dendrites receive them.

Neurotransmitters are chemical messengers that help generate the electrical signals that are sent from one neuron to another. They enable the communication between neurons that is crucial to our mental and emotional states, including depression, anxiety, motivation, and pleasure.

This complex communication system is continually producing sensations and emotions within us. Every moment, sensory information from our environment is streaming into our bodies. This could be the warmth of the sun on our skin, the aroma of a flower, or the sound of a favorite song.

Once the body registers these experiences, they're directed to the brain, which processes and interprets this information, determining the appropriate response. For example, if we bite into a lemon, the sensory information travels to the brain, which interprets the taste as 'sour,' triggering a reaction like puckering our lips or squinting our eyes.

But it's not just about physical sensations. This system also plays a crucial role in our emotional responses. The brain interprets sensory information and attaches emotions, creating our emotional reactions to the world around us. So, the smell of a particular perfume might not just be interpreted as 'sweet' or 'floral', but could also trigger feelings of happiness or nostalgia if it's associated with a happy memory.

In this way, our brain continually interprets sensory information and orchestrates physical and emotional responses, creating our rich tapestry of experiences and reactions.

Now, let's zoom in on a few key players that help generate these emotional and physical responses. The following neurotransmitters each have a unique role in our mental health:

- **Dopamine** motivates us by rewarding us with pleasurable sensations. When dopamine levels are too high or too low, it can lead to mental health issues, such as depression, attention-deficit hyperactivity disorder (ADIID), and anxiety.

- **Serotonin** helps stabilize our mood. It is also involved in sleep patterns, digestion, and general feelings of well-being. Low serotonin levels are often associated with depression and anxiety.

- **Norepinephrine** allows us to focus, and regulates heart rate, blood pressure, and stress levels. Low levels of norepinephrine can lead to low energy levels, fatigue, and difficulty concentrating.

- **GABA** is crucial for sleep and relaxation, helping us combat stress. Low GABA levels can result in a restless night, muscle tension, and anxiety.

- **Glutamate** is involved in learning and memory. Low levels of glutamate can lead to confusion and difficulty focusing and learning.

By understanding the roles these neurotransmitters play in mental health, we can better use food to increase their availability depending on what symptoms we are targeting. For instance, foods rich in tyrosine, such as almonds, bananas, and avocados, can boost dopamine levels, while foods high in magnesium, like leafy greens and legumes, can help increase GABA levels.

While the neurobiology of our brain plays a central role in our mental well-being, another fascinating world within our bodies also contributes to this process. Let's now turn our attention to the bustling community of microscopic critters we host.

Microbiota

Our microbiome is a diverse collection of trillions of bacteria, fungi, and viruses, collectively known as microbiota, that coexist in the nooks and crannies of our bodies. They can be found in our intestinal tract, skin, mouth, and nasal cavities, forming a complex and interdependent ecosystem. They're hard at work, contributing to our health and well-being in ways we're only beginning to understand.

While some might view bacteria and viruses with suspicion, it's essential to recognize that many of these microorganisms are beneficial. Some are responsible for producing vitamins, while others produce hormones and neurotransmitters. There are even certain viruses in our gut that interact with bacteria in ways that are advantageous to us. It's a delicate balance, with each microorganism playing its part in the grand scheme of our health.

Emerging research suggests that our microbiota might be conducting more than just our physical health. They could also be orchestrating our mental health, pulling the strings on our mood. But how well they do this is based on the overall health of the gut microbiome.

A healthy gut microbiome is characterized by a

diverse and harmonious community of microbial species, each performing its unique role to maintain equilibrium. This balance is crucial for warding off harmful pathogens and ensuring our bodies operate optimally.

Various factors, including diet, genetics, lifestyle, and the environment, influence the state of our microbiome. A nutritious diet rich in fresh fruits, vegetables, nuts, seeds, legumes, and whole grains helps foster a robust microbiome. Incorporating fermented foods offers a regular supply of beneficial bacteria to the community. Exercise and stress management further support our microbes. And when our microbiome is happy our mood follows suit.

In a 2022 study[4], the relationship between gut microbiota and depression symptoms was evaluated in 1,133 participants. They discovered that certain microbial species (Eggerthella, Coprococcus, and others) were associated with depression. Most of these bacteria were found in reduced amounts in individuals with depression, while a few were increased. Notably, bacteria from the Eggerthella genus were linked to heightened depression symptoms. The study suggests that these bacteria play a role in producing neurotransmitters like glutamate, butyrate, serotonin, and GABA, which may influence depression symptoms. This is one of many studies shedding light on the profound connection between our microbiota and mental health.

So, the next time you're feeling low, remember you've

---

[4] https://pubmed.ncbi.nlm.nih.gov/29064009/

got trillions of microscopic friends ready to help. By eating a healthy diet, introducing fermented foods, exercising, and managing stress, you're not only taking care of yourself; you're taking care of your microbiota. And in return, they'll do their part to care for you.

The fascinating interplay between our microbiota and mental health is just one part of the mood-food connection. As we further explore this relationship, we'll head out along the communication superhighway where much of the action occurs.

Gut-Brain Axis

The Gut-Brain Axis is an intricate communication network between our digestive system and brain. The communication here is a dynamic, ongoing dialogue that profoundly impacts our physical and mental health.

Our digestive system, with its vast network of neurons, is often referred to as our 'second brain.' This is because it has its own independent neural system that communicates directly with our central nervous system. While our body's enzymes metabolize food, our gut microorganisms play a crucial role in breaking down certain substances and influencing the production of beneficial compounds like neurotransmitters. These molecules, once absorbed by the intestinal walls, travel through our bloodstream, influencing various bodily functions, from brain activity and mood regulation to immune responses.

Yet, it's not just the digestive system doing all the talking. The brain is busy dispatching its own set of signals and neurotransmitters to the digestive system. Depending on the nature of these signals, our gut might experience changes in motility, secretion, or even immune responses, showcasing the profound interconnectedness of these two systems.

The vagus nerve is at the heart of this communication network, a direct line running from the digestive system to the brain stem. This nerve allows for the two-way communication. It's the express delivery service of the Gut-Brain Axis.

The Gut-Brain Axis plays a crucial role in mental health. An imbalance in the gut can lead to an imbalance in the types of hormones and neurotransmitters sent to the brain, which may result in higher levels of anxiety, depression, or other mental health issues.

The importance of this two-way communication, the neurotransmitters produced, and the vagus nerve's role cannot be overstated. It's a testament to the powerful connection between the body and the brain, a connection we're only beginning to understand.

You now have a basic understanding of the intricate components that make up this remarkable system. But to function at its best, it requires regular input derived from our diet. In the following sections, we'll explore how plants and their array of nutrients serve as an excellent source for this vital input.

Plants

Let's take a moment to marvel at the sheer variety of edible plants available to us. There are about 200,000 different nutrient-dense, fiber-rich, gut-friendly options.[5] And with innovative chefs and food bloggers constantly churning out creative new recipes, you won't get bored with a plant-based diet!

As mentioned before, our gut is home to trillions of bacteria, forming a complex ecosystem. In this bustling metropolis, the thousands of different bacterial strains each have a preferred diet that will allow them to perform their duties well.

To keep this diverse workforce happy and productive, we need to provide a variety of plant-based foods. In his book *Fiber Fueled*, Dr. Bulsiewicz suggests that the diversity of plants in your diet is the greatest predictor of a healthy gut microbiome. By mindfully choosing a variety of plants we essentialy provide a well-stocked pantry for our gut bacteria, allowing them to thrive on a smorgasbord of nutrients. These nutrients include dietary fiber, prebiotics, and phytonutrients.

---

[5] https://www.weforum.org/agenda/2016/01/why-do-we-consume-only-a-tiny-fraction-of-the-world-s-edible-plants

Within the gut microbiome, each distinct microbe plays a different role in our health. So, we benefit from having a diverse makeup of these helpful critters. The U.S. Gut Project analyzed feces samples from over 10,000 citizen scientists worldwide, providing valuable insights into our intestinal microbe differences. This study found that those consuming at least 30 different plant-based foods per week had a much greater diversity of gut microbes compared to those eating fewer than 10. Moreover, those eating the 30 plants a week also reduced symptoms of dysbiosis.[6]

To get 30 plants a week, we can incorporate whole foods from these four main categories:

- **Legumes**, such as lentils, chickpeas, black beans, and peas, are packed with protein, fiber, and various vitamins and minerals.

- **Nuts and seeds**, such as almonds, walnuts, flaxseeds, and chia seeds, are rich in healthy fats, fiber, and antioxidants, providing essential nutrients for upkeep and repair.

- **Fruits and vegetables**, like apples, carrots, bell peppers, spinach, blueberries, and eggplants contain fiber and are loaded with phytonutrients.

---

[6] https://pubmed.ncbi.nlm.nih.gov/29795809/

- **Whole grains**, like brown rice, quinoa, oats, and whole wheat bread, are rich in dietary fiber, nourishing gut bacteria. They also contain B vitamins, iron, folate, selenium, potassium, and magnesium, all essential for mental health.

A diet that includes a variety of foods from each of these categories helps support a thriving, healthy gut microbiome. And as you know by now, this can have a significant impact on how you feel on many levels. So, next time you're at the grocery store, consider adding a colorful variety of plant-based foods to your cart. Your microbiome will thank you.

Next, let's look at a few of the components plants offer us to support our mental and emotional health.

Macronutrients

Macronutrients, namely carbohydrates, proteins, and fats, are the nutritional powerhouses that fuel our bodies. They each play distinct roles: carbohydrates, including fiber, provide quick energy and regulate digestion; proteins contribute to structure, repair, and the creation of neurotransmitters; and fats ensure long-term energy storage and support vital functions. Balancing these macronutrients in your diet is key to maintaining good health and promoting mental well-being.

Carbohydrates

Carbohydrates (carbs), often misunderstood and sometimes maligned, play a vital role in our overall well-being, particularly in mental health. The key lies in understanding the difference between simple and complex carbs and their impact on our body and mind.

Complex carbs are found in whole grains like brown rice, quinoa, whole wheat bread, and fruits and vegetables. These nutrient-dense foods not only provide essential energy but also support mental well-being.

Unlike simple carbs, which can cause rapid spikes and drops in blood sugar levels, complex carbohydrates provide a slow and steady release of glucose. This controlled release is due to fiber, which helps slow the digestion of these nutrients.

The importance of this slow release cannot be overstated, especially when it comes to mental health. Rapid spikes in blood sugar can lead to anxiety and irritability, while the subsequent drop can cause fatigue and depression. Complex carbs help avoid this rollercoaster effect, supporting a more balanced and stable mood.

In addition, carbohydrates have an indirect role in the

production of neurotransmitters like serotonin. When we consume carbs, our bodies release insulin. This insulin response facilitates the transport of amino acids like tryptophan into the brain. Once inside the brain, tryptophan can be converted into serotonin. Complex carbs, due to their slower digestion and absorption rates, can lead to a more gradual and sustained insulin response. This potentially supports a consistent influx of tryptophan into the brain, thereby aiding in the steady synthesis of serotonin. In essence, complex carbohydrates contribute to our overall mental health by indirectly supporting the production of key neurotransmitters.

Complex carbohydrates are more than just fuel for our bodies. They are integral to our mental health, providing steady energy, supporting neurotransmitter production, and contributing to gut health (discussed next, in the section on fiber). By making mindful choices and focusing on whole grains, fruits, and vegetables, we can nourish both our bodies and minds.

Fiber

We are all googly-eyed over protein. In health and fitness circles, we are often asked, "Did you get your protein today?" Though it is a necessary component in nutrition, it has been over-hyped. And while protein basks in the lime lite, poor ol' fiber is working away in the background, scrubbing our insides clean and feeding the often fiber-starved microorganisms in our gut.

Mostly we know fiber as a way to keep us "regular." When blocked up, we're told to eat prunes, the fiber in them helping to move things along. And while this is one of the thankless jobs these carbohydrates undertake, we don't often hear about the other role for which we should be singing their praises.

We aren't focused on fiber because most of the action happens "down there." And this is about as "down there" as we can get since we are talking about the large intestine and colon. The microbes in the small intestine aren't very considerate of their brethren further down the tubes; they are happy enough to gobble up all the protein and fats while leaving the more tricky-to-digest fiber for the hungry critters below.

And, because the Western diet is pathetically deficient

in fiber, the microbes in our lower digestive tract leave quite disappointed every time they gather for a meal.

Fiber is an essential component of having a healthy and balanced gut microbiome. It acts as fuel for beneficial microorganisms, providing them with energy. Consisting of long-chain carbohydrates, fiber needs a large amount of bacterial fermentation to break it down into smaller molecules. This fermentation process allows these bacteria to extract energy, creating short-chain fatty acids (SCFAs) used in the digestive process. SCFAs tell the immune cells in our gut what jobs to take on, supporting the body's defense mechanisms. The presence of these SCFAs can have various health-promoting effects, including reducing inflammation and protecting our gut against dysbiosis.

Plant foods are the primary source of dietary fiber, offering a range of fiber types from the many foods within the plant kingdom. By diversifying our intake of plant-based foods, we nurture our gut microbiome with varied fibers.

Here's a quick break-down of some of the best options for high-fiber plant foods:

- **Barley**: Contains both soluble and insoluble fiber

- **Quinoa**: A gluten-free grain that's high in fiber

- **Brown Rice**: Offers more fiber than its white counterpart.

- **Wheat Bran**: A byproduct of wheat milling, it's a great source of insoluble fiber.

- **Raspberries**: Among the highest-fiber fruits.

- **Chia Seeds**: These tiny seeds expand in the stomach, helping to keep you full.

- **Almonds**: A nut high in fiber and healthy fats.

- **Flaxseeds**: Best consumed ground for better nutrient absorption.

- **Broccoli**: Contains both soluble and insoluble fiber.

- **Brussels Sprouts**: A cruciferous vegetable that's a good source of fiber.

- **Carrots**: A root vegetable that's versatile and high in fiber.

- **Pears**: Especially with the skin on.

- **Avocado**: Contains soluble and insoluble fiber.

- **Oranges**: Offer a good amount of fiber and vitamin C.

- **Popcorn**: A whole grain and a good source of fiber.

- **Sweet Potatoes**: Especially with the skin on.

- **Spinach and other Leafy Greens**: While not as high in fiber as some other foods on this list, they still contribute to daily fiber intake.

Prebiotics, a special form of dietary fiber, deserve a spotlight in this fiber narrative. While all prebiotics are fiber, not all fibers are prebiotics. Prebiotics resist digestion in the upper part of the gastrointestinal tract and are fermented by the gut microbes in the colon. Foods rich in prebiotics specifically nourish and stimulate the growth of beneficial bacteria. By feeding on these prebiotics, the beneficial bacteria produce the aforementioned SCFAs, further enhancing gut health and, by extension, mental well-being. In essence, while fiber provides a broad spectrum of benefits to our gut microbiome, prebiotics target and boost the health-promoting bacteria, ensuring a harmonious gut environment.

Incorporating these prebiotic-rich foods into our diet ensures that gut bacteria in the colon have the specific nourishment they need to thrive:

- **Apples**: They contain pectin, a type of soluble fiber that acts as a prebiotic.

- **Asparagus**: Contains inulin, a type of soluble fiber that serves as a prebiotic.

- **Bananas**: Especially unripe bananas, are a source of resistant starch, a type of prebiotic fiber.

- **Garlic**: Contains fructooligosaccharides (FOS), which serve as prebiotics.

- **Legumes** (chickpeas, kidney beans, lentils, soybeans): They are rich in fibers and resistant starch, both of which have prebiotic properties.

- **Oats**: Contain beta-glucans and resistant starch, both of which have prebiotic effects.

- **Onions** (leeks, shallots, and spring onions, too): Like garlic, they contain fructooligosaccharides (FOS).

- **Savoy Cabbage**: Contains various fibers that can act as prebiotics.

- **Seaweed**: Some studies suggest that seaweed can act as a prebiotic.

As previously mentioned, having a balanced gut microbiome is essential for mental health, as it plays a significant role in neurotransmitter production. As these microbes ferment the fibers, the SCFAs they produce can cross the blood-brain barrier, fueling the creation of neurotransmitters such as serotonin and dopamine.

The average daily fiber intake for adults in many

modern societies hovers around a mere 15 grams[7], falling significantly short of the recommended 25-35 grams. But, even this recommendation is quite low. Aiming for an intake of 38-50 grams of fiber daily can vastly improve gut health. This target is not as ambitious as it might seem when we consider the dietary habits of traditional populations. For instance, those following a traditional hunter-gatherer lifestyle, such as the Hadza of Tanzania, have been known to consume upwards of 100 grams of fiber per day.[8] By striving for a daily intake of 38-50 grams, we're not only aligning with the practices of populations known for their robust health but also taking a proactive step towards enhancing our own well-being.

As you can see, fiber plays a pivotal role in the balance of our gut microbiome. Through its fermentation, it provides energy to microorganisms within the gut, which are essential for the production of health-promoting metabolites. This, in turn, provides for a balanced and diversified gut microbiome, which is beneficial for mental health due to the production of neurotransmitters.

So, the question we should be asking is, "Did you get your fiber today?" Did you? If not, you might consider making this your first goal in this process.

---

[7] https://www.health.harvard.edu/blog/should-i-be-eating-more-fiber-2019022115927
[8] https://stanmed.stanford.edu/hunter-gatherer-diets-offer-clues-to-gut-bug-diversity/

Proteins

Proteins are fundamental to our physical well-being, but their role extends far beyond muscle building and tissue repair. They are essential players in our mental health, influencing everything from mood regulation to mental focus.

Amino acids are the building blocks of proteins and are necessary to form neurotransmitters. Our bodies can synthesize eleven of the twenty amino acids, but the other nine must come from our diet. Since neurotransmitters help regulate mood, stress levels, sex drive, and sleep-wake cycles, it is important to get the full range of amino acids.

When we consume protein-rich foods, our bodies first use these proteins for growth and repair. The leftover amino acids can then be used to manufacture neurotransmitters, stored in vesicles, and released as needed.

In the Western diet, we often get it backward when balancing our carbohydrate and protein intake. Breakfasts are frequently carb-heavy with items like bagels and cereals, while dinners lean more towards proteins, often with meat as the main focus. However, this pattern might not be the most beneficial for those aiming to maintain focus and alertness throughout the day.

Starting with a breakfast dominated by simple carbs can lead to mental fatigue due to the rapid energy surge followed by a swift decline, leaving us feeling foggy and unfocused. In contrast, meals balanced with complex carbs and high protein offer a slow and steady energy release, promoting mental clarity. Getting enough protein can help our body synthesize norepinephrine, a neurotransmitter crucial to concentration and alertness. By prioritizing protein in the morning and early afternoon, we can support our brain's ability to function optimally throughout the day.

Here are some plant-based sources of complete proteins with all nine essential amino acids:

- **Soybeans and Soy Products**: In addition to tofu, other soy products like tempeh and edamame are complete proteins.

- **Buckwheat**: Despite its name, buckwheat is not related to wheat and is gluten-free. It can be found in products like buckwheat noodles and kasha.

- **Hemp Seeds**: These seeds can be consumed whole or as hemp protein powder.

- **Chia Seeds**: Besides being a complete protein, these seeds are also rich in omega-3 fatty acids. Chia seed pudding is a great way to start the day!

- **Nutritional Yeast**: Often used for its cheesy flavor in vegan dishes, it's packed with B-vitamins.

- **Spirulina**: This blue-green algae is often found in supplement form or added to smoothies.

- **Amaranth**: A nutrient-dense grain, amaranth is rich in fiber, vitamins, minerals, and antioxidants.

- **Teff**: This tiny grain is native to Ethiopia and is a versatile grain that can be used in a variety of dishes.

- **Quinoa**: Known for its nutty flavor and unique texture, quinoa is a versatile grain that's high in fiber and various essential nutrients, often used as a substitute for rice or pasta.

If you aren't consuming complete-protein foods daily, combining other protein-rich whole foods to get the full set of amino acids, is vital. We'll provide some examples of easy combos in the tips and tricks section of this book.

Incorporating a variety of protein-rich plant-based foods ensures access to the essential amino acids necessary for mental well-being. By making mindful choices in our protein consumption, we can support not only our physical health but our mental and emotional wellness.

Fats

Your brain is fat. I'm not trying to put you down. Mine is too, and that's a good thing; they're supposed to be. Our brains are mostly fat, composed of 60% fat, in fact. They are the fattest organ in the body. Since much of the fats we consume end up here, we should think twice about the fats we put into our bodies.

As mentioned before, neurotransmitters are the chemical messages expressed as feelings, desires, pleasure, movement, and many other human functions. So, ensuring these messages get relayed correctly is essential, and this is where fat comes in.

As messages travel from one cell to the next, jumping from one cell's axon to another cell's dendrite, these messages need to be contained within the targeted range. This is achieved by coating the system with a myelin sheath made of fat. Think of it as the casing on an electrical cord.

Consider this scenario: a squirrel gets into the attic of your home and chews a hole in your wiring—nibbling right through the plastic coating—allowing electrical currents to spill out all over the place. You flip your light switch (presuming you still have a light switch, and your house hasn't burned to the ground), and: no light. The message is not being received.

The same thing can happen when our myelin sheath gets damaged. This is part of the problem for people suffering from multiple sclerosis (MS). They have trouble with mobility because the message that was supposed to tell the leg to make a specific movement never fully reached the leg.

Things like excessive alcohol use and an unhealthy diet can cause these fatty coatings to become rigid and crack, allowing messages to seep out. On the other hand, a healthy diet with the right amount of fat contributes to smoother communication between cells.

We don't like to judge around here, but when it comes to fats, we will: there are good and bad fats. The Standard American Diet (SAD) contains more of the latter. This is because diets loaded with fried foods, baked goods, processed snacks, and animal-based foods contain large amounts of trans and saturated fats. These not only contribute to cardiovascular disease but can also impact our mental health. Excessive intake of these unhealthy fats can lead to inflammation and oxidative stress, which are linked to depression and anxiety.

The "good" fats are monounsaturated and polyunsaturated fats, which include omega-6 and omega-3 fatty acids. While we need both, the typical Western diet often contains too much omega-6s from fried and processed foods and insufficient omega-3s.

Omega-3 fatty acids are important for brain development and can help protect against depression[9] and anxiety.[10] They also have anti-inflammatory properties and play an important role in cognitive and memory functions.

Aiming for a balanced ratio of omega-6s to omega-3s is crucial for optimal health. The ideal target is a ratio between 1:1 to 3:1 (omega-6: omega-3). This is not far from the dietary patterns of our ancestors; traditional hunter-gatherer diets typically maintained a 1:1 ratio. In contrast, the Japanese diet, often praised for its health benefits, has a ratio of 4:1. Alarmingly, SAD skews this balance dramatically, with ratios ranging from 20:1 to 25:1. By striving to emulate the balanced intake of traditional diets, we can move closer to a nutritional profile that supports overall well-being.

To balance the ratio and reduce the inflammatory impact of an excess of omega-6, we need to choose food sources of omega-3. Lucky for us, there are some wonderful plant-based foods high in omega-3s, like flaxseeds, chia seeds, walnuts, and dark green leafy vegetables—though to a lesser degree.

Not so lucky for us, a balanced diet requires three forms of omega-3—ALA, EPA, and DHA—though plant-based foods primarily contain ALA. Each form plays a crucial role in supporting heart and brain function, as well as reducing inflammation. While ALA can be converted into EPA and DHA, the conversion

---

[9] https://pubmed.ncbi.nlm.nih.gov/24805797/
[10] https://www.ncbi.nlm.nih.gov/pmc/articles/
PMC6324500/

process in humans is relatively inefficient. Factors such as age, gender, and an adequate intake of specific vitamins and minerals impact the efficiency of this conversion. Ensuring a sufficient intake of vitamins B3, B6, and C, as well as zinc and magnesium, is necessary for this conversion process to occur.

When we hear about getting our omega-3s, we are often told that we need more fatty fish in our diets, fish being a source of all three forms of omega-3s. Some people may point to this as one of the reasons why a vegan diet is inadequate.

But fish wouldn't have these forms of omega-3s if it weren't for plants. Fish accumulate EPA and DHA in their tissues by consuming microalgae. Farmed fish are often fed fishmeal and fish oil obtained from wild-caught fish that contain EPA and DHA. But we don't need fish to get these forms of omega-3s as we can go right to the source by taking plant-based algae supplements that already contain them.

The fats we consume play a crucial role in our brain health and function. They form the protective myelin sheath that ensures the smooth transmission of messages between cells, influencing our feelings, desires, and movements. While unhealthy fats from processed foods can damage this system, "good" fats, particularly omega-3 fatty acids, support brain development and protect against inflammation and oxidative stresss. We can nourish our brains and promote optimal mental health by choosing plant-based sources of these beneficial fats.

Micronutrients

Micronutrients, including essential vitamins and minerals, are the subtle yet powerful conductors behind the scenes of our health. Despite being required in smaller amounts than macronutrients, their impact on our bodies and minds is profound. They support a range of functions, from brain health to guiding the chemical reactions within our cells and forming the structure of our bones and teeth. They also ensure the proper function of our heart and muscles. Furthermore, micronutrients play a role in regulating mood, sleep, and libido and help us manage stress.

Despite their small requirements, a deficiency in any of these micronutrients can lead to significant health problems. So, eating a range of plants and supplementing where needed is the best way to ensure you get all the micronutrients your body needs to stay healthy and function optimally.

Vitamins

In the realm of mental health, vitamins play a crucial role. Here, we'll explore some of the key players: B vitamins and vitamins C, D, and E.

Water-soluble and fat-soluble vitamins differ in how they are absorbed, stored, and excreted by the body. Water-soluble vitamins, which include all the B vitamins and vitamin C, are absorbed directly into the bloodstream during digestion. They are not stored in large amounts in the body, and any excess is excreted through urine. This means they must be consumed more regularly, often daily, to maintain adequate levels.

Fat-soluble vitamins, which include vitamins A, D, and E, are absorbed in the intestines along with dietary fat and then stored in the liver and fatty tissues. Because they are stored in the body, they do not necessarily need to be consumed every day. But, it also means they can accumulate and reach toxic levels if consumed in large amounts over time. So, it's important to stay within the recommended amounts of these vitamins.

B vitamins, often called the 'anti-stress vitamins,' are integral to our mental health. They are essential for healthy brain function and are critical components in the synthesis of neurotransmitters that regulate things like mood, sleep, and sex drive. Studies have shown that people who ate foods high in B vitamins had better depression, anxiety, and stress scores.[11] A deficiency in B vitamins can also lead to fatigue and irritability.

Vitamin B1, or Thiamine, is a catalyst in converting glucose into energy, a process vital for producing GABA. This neurotransmitter helps control fear and anxiety when neurons become overexcited. B1 also helps metabolize the neurotransmitter acetylcholine, which is important for mental alertness, attention, and focus. Finally, B1 assists in the metabolism of tryptophan into serotonin. Alcoholism and anorexia can impair thiamine levels. Tea, coffee, and shellfish can also impair its absorption. Nuts, seeds, legumes, and whole grains are excellent sources of B1.

Vitamin B2, or Riboflavin, is necessary to synthesize other B vitamins (B3, B6, B9, B12) that are critical for a healthy mood. Some studies have found evidence that suggests B2 can help prevent depression and anxiety[12]. Excessive alcohol can cause B2 deficiency. Good sources of B2 include mushrooms, almonds, leafy greens, legumes, and broccoli.

Vitamin B3, or Niacin, helps maintain the body's cells, is a powerful antioxidant, and is essential for

---

[11] https://www.ncbi.nlm.nih.gov/pmc/articles/ PMC6770181/
[12] https://www.ncbi.nlm.nih.gov/pmc/articles/ PMC10060244/

metabolism and neuronal function. B3 also helps make sex hormones and improves circulation, which impacts sexual performance. Good sources of B3 are mushrooms, nuts and seeds, sun-dried tomatoes, avocado, and dates.

B5, or Pantothenic Acid, helps us convert protein and fat into energy. It is also needed for the uptake of amino acids (which we use to manufacture neurotransmitters) and acetylcholine. B5 can also help with stress reduction and anxiety management. Adrenal glands need B5 to help produce the stress hormone cortisol as well. Foods like whole grains, broccoli, peanuts, mushrooms, and sweet potatoes are rich in B5.

Vitamin B6, or Pyridoxine, is a co-factor for the enzyme that converts glutamate into GABA and tryptophan into serotonin. It also aids in producing dopamine. B6 helps regulate the body's melatonin levels, influencing sleep cycles. B6 may also help reduce mental fatigue by improving circulation and oxygenation to the brain. Some of the best sources of vitamin B6 include legumes (especially black beans, lentils, and chickpeas), nuts and seeds, dark leafy greens, avocados, sweet potatoes, potatoes, and bananas.

Vitamin B9, or Folate, aids in the conversion of precursors into their active forms, thereby facilitating the production of serotonin, dopamine, norepinephrine, and GABA. It also helps reduce homocysteine levels. High homocysteine levels have been linked to an increased risk of depression.[13] B9 helps synthesize brain-derived neurotrophic factor (BDNF), essential for neural plasticity. Finally, B9 is involved in melatonin production, helping improve sleep. Foods such as dark leafy greens, asparagus, broccoli, legumes, avocados, and citrus fruits are excellent sources of B9.

Vitamin B12 is necessary for the functioning of the nervous system and helps the body produce dopamine. It is mostly found in animal products and deficiency is common. So vegans and individuals on a plant-based diet should take it in supplement form.

Vitamin C is an essential nutrient for synthesizing neurotransmitters like dopamine, noradrenaline, and serotonin. Some studies have shown that it may improve symptoms in mood and stress-related disorders.[14] Vitamin C is a powerful antioxidant that helps reduce inflammation. Plant foods rich in Vitamin C include bell peppers, kiwifruit, broccoli, oranges, and strawberries.

Vitamin A, crucial for brain health and cognitive function, is associated with reduced depression, anxiety, and stress levels. It protects brain cells in key emotional areas and has antioxidant properties that can lessen inflammation, often linked to mental health issues. Additionally, vitamin A plays a role in

---

[13] https://www.ncbi.nlm.nih.gov/pmc/articles/ PMC8372975/
[14] https://www.sciencedirect.com/science/article/pii/ S0955286320304915

developing the central nervous system and regulating sleep. Deficiency is rare but can occur in conditions affecting digestion, like celiac disease, or alcoholism. Rich sources of vitamin A include sweet potatoes, carrots, kale, spinach, and pumpkin seeds.

Vitamin D, often called the 'sunshine vitamin,' is crucial for mood regulation and cognitive function. It is synthesized in our skin in response to sunlight. Despite also being available in many fortified foods, deficiency is common; we don't get outside enough. When consuming a plant-based diet, besides fortified foods like some plant-based milks and cereals, mushrooms exposed to UV light are the only plant-based source of Vitamin D. As a result, taking a supplement is recommended.

Vitamin E, a potent antioxidant, protects our cells from damage and is involved in the regulation of mental function and mood. You can find high levels of Vitamin E in sunflower seeds, almonds, Swiss chard, avocado, and spinach.

It's important to remember that the vitamins discussed do not operate in isolation. Often, they act synergistically, enhancing each other's bioavailability. For example, Vitamin B6 is necessary for the effective uptake of Vitamin B12. Similarly, Vitamin D plays a crucial role in enhancing the absorption of minerals such as calcium and phosphorus.

Some medications, excessive intake of caffeine or alcohol, and certain health conditions can inhibit the absorption of these vitamins. So, it is important to consume a balanced diet that includes a variety of foods rich in these vitamins and be mindful when using certain substances.

In this brief overview, you can see how each vitamin plays a pivotal role in our mental health. Their roles range from synthesizing neurotransmitters and acting as antioxidants to supporting our brain and nervous system. Therefore, ensuring an adequate intake of these vitamins as well as the minerals we'll discuss in the next section is crucial for optimal mental and emotional wellness.

Minerals

Minerals are another essential nutrient that can support our mental health. This section will focus on four key minerals: iron, magnesium, selenium, and zinc. Each of these minerals uniquely supports our mental well-being, affecting our mood and cognitive function.

Iron is a crucial mineral that our bodies need for optimal functioning. It plays a vital role in producing hemoglobin, a protein that allows red blood cells to carry oxygen to all parts of the body. It also plays a significant role in maintaining healthy skin, hair, and nails.

Iron plays a vital role in mental health, being integral in the production of various neurotransmitters such as dopamine, norepinephrine, and serotonin. It is crucial for cognitive development and function. Studies[15] indicate that iron deficiency during infancy and childhood can lead to significant cognitive and behavioral issues, including developmental delays, learning difficulties, and diminished cognitive performance in adulthood. Furthermore, iron deficiency has been associated with mental health

---

[15] https://www.ncbi.nlm.nih.gov/pmc/articles/ PMC1540447/

conditions like depression, anxiety, and sleep disorders University of Michigan Department of Psychiatry.[16]

Additionally, the absorption of iron is influenced by various factors. Vitamin C is known to enhance iron absorption, while substances like phytates (found in grains and legumes) and polyphenols (present in some vegetables and tea) can inhibit it. Therefore, consuming iron-rich foods like spinach alongside a source of vitamin C, such as citrus fruits, is an effective way to boost iron absorption in the body.

Plant-based sources of iron include lentils, chickpeas, beans, tofu, cashew nuts, chia seeds, flaxseed, hemp seeds, pumpkin seeds, kale, dried apricots and figs, raisins, and quinoa.

Magnesium is another essential mineral that plays a role in over 300 enzymatic reactions within the body, including the metabolism of food, synthesis of fatty acids and proteins, and the transmission of nerve impulses.

The body needs magnesium for the health of the nervous system and brain function. It is involved in synthesizing neurotransmitters, including serotonin. Low levels of magnesium have been linked to an increased risk for anxiety and depression. It also plays a role in maintaining healthy sleep patterns and

---

[16] https://medicine.umich.edu/dept/psychiatry/news/archive/202305/could-low-iron-be-making-your-mental-health-symptoms-worse#

regulates the body's stress-response system.

Magnesium is found in various plant-based foods, including legumes, nuts, seeds, whole grains, and green leafy vegetables. Other good sources include avocados, bananas, and dark chocolate.

Selenium is a trace mineral that is essential for good health. It is important for cognitive function, a healthy immune system, and fertility in both men and women.

Selenium plays a critical role in the health of your brain. It is involved in the production of antioxidants that protect neurons from damage. It also has anti-inflammatory properties, which can help reduce inflammation in the brain.

A selenium deficiency can lead to cognitive decline and neurological diseases such as Alzheimer's and Parkinson's. Low levels can also interfere with the normal conversion of ALA into EPA and DHA omega-3s. On the other hand, a diet rich in selenium can improve mood and reduce anxiety.

Plant-based sources of selenium include Brazil nuts, sunflower seeds, whole grains, and mushrooms.

Zinc is crucial for metabolism, immune function, and cell repair. It also plays a role in maintaining a healthy brain and mental function.

Zinc is involved in the structure and function of the brain, and it plays a key role in neurotransmitter function and helps maintain the brain's defense system. Zinc deficiency can lead to changes in behavior, reduced learning ability, and decreased mental function.

Zinc also helps with mood regulation. Low levels of have been linked to anxiety and depression.[17]

Zinc absorption is better from animal sources, but there are still plenty of plant-based sources, including whole grains, wheat germ, tofu, sprouted bread, legumes, nuts, and seeds.

While these minerals are essential for optimal mental health, it's important to maintain a balanced diet and not to consume them in excess. If deficient, and supplementation is needed, it can be helpful to consult with a healthcare professional before starting a new regimen. And, though it can be tempting to get your vitamins and minerals by simply taking a pill, by doing so, you are missing out on some of the benefits that plants offer, namely fiber and the range of phytochemicals that we will explore in the next section.

---

[17] https://psychcentral.com/health/zinc-anxiety#zinc-and-anxiety

Phytochemicals

The terms "phytochemicals" and "phytonutrients" are often used interchangeably, and the distinction between them can be somewhat blurred. Both are natural compounds only found in plants that protect the plant against pests, diseases, and UV radiation. They are not technically micronutrients, as they aren't deemed essential for human health. However, they can be profoundly useful.

Phytonutrients are a subset of phytochemicals, specifically those known or believed to benefit human health. Many of them protect the body from oxidative stress and inflammation, while also counteracting harmful effects associated with poor nutrition, environmental toxins, aging, chronic diseases, and immune system imbalances.

There are several major classes of phytonutrients, each with its unique characteristics and functions:

Flavonoids:
- Subclasses include anthocyanins, flavones, isoflavones, flavanones, flavonols, and catechins.
- Found in fruits, vegetables, tea, and wine.
- Known for antioxidant, anti-inflammatory, and heart health benefits.

- Catechins, found in green tea, may have a positive impact on mood and cognitive function.
- Isoflavones, found in soy, may have a positive impact on mood, particularly in postmenopausal women.
- Luteolin is a type of flavone found in foods such as celery, broccoli, artichokes, peppermint, green pepper, parsley, thyme, olives, and carrots. Researchers propose that luteolin may help decrease brain fog by reducing inflammation in the brain, limiting oxidative stress, inhibiting the activity of viruses, and reducing cognitive decline.
- Anthocyanins are responsible for the deep red, blue, and purple pigments found in many berries. They have been studied for their potential benefits in heart health, brain function, and anti-inflammatory effects.
- Quercetin is a type a flavonol found in many berries, including cranberries and blueberries. It has been studied for its potential anti-allergic, anti-cancer, and anti-inflammatory properties. It may help with stress and anxiety, too.

Carotenoids:
- Subclasses include beta-carotene, lycopene, lutein, and zeaxanthin.
- Found in red, orange, yellow, and green fruits and vegetables.
- Important for eye health, immune function, and skin health.
- Lutein and Zeaxanthin, found in leafy greens, may support cognitive function and reduce the risk of mental decline with aging.

Glucosinolates:
- Found in cruciferous vegetables like broccoli, cabbage, and kale.
- Studied for potential anti-cancer properties.

Saponins:
- Found in beans and legumes.
- May have immune-boosting and cholesterol-lowering effects.
- May also support mental health through antioxidant and anti-inflammatory effects.

Lignans:
- Found in seeds, grains, and vegetables.
- Have antioxidant properties and may contribute to heart health.

Tannins:
- Found in tea, coffee, and some fruits.
- Known for astringent properties and potential digestive health benefits.

Alkaloids:
- Found in tomatoes, potatoes, and peppers.
- Have various effects on human health, some beneficial and some potentially harmful.

Phenolic Acids:
- Subclasses include stilbenes (like resveratrol) and ellagic acid.
- Found in berries, grapes, and whole grains.
- Have antioxidant and anti-inflammatory effects.
- Resveratrol, found in red wine and grapes, has been studied for potential neuroprotective

effects.

Terpenes:
- Include monoterpenes, sesquiterpenes, and diterpenes.
- Found in herbs and citrus fruits.
- May have anti-cancer and anti-inflammatory properties.

Organosulfur Compounds:
- Found in garlic, onions, and leeks.
- May have anti-cancer and heart health benefits.

Polyphenols are a diverse group of phytonutrients found in many plant foods. Of the phytonutrient classes listed above, flavonoids, phenolic acids, tannins, and lignans are all considered polyphenols.

Polyphenols are a type of antioxidant known to counteract oxidative stress by neutralizing free radicals. By mitigating oxidative stress, antioxidants can reduce excessive inflammatory responses in the body. This is important because chronic inflammation is increasingly being recognized as a potential contributor to various mental health conditions, including depression, mental decline, and possibly anxiety.[18]

In general, many foods that are darker in color are higher in antioxidants. The deep colors of many fruits, vegetables, and other foods often come from compounds such as anthocyanins, carotenoids, and

---

[18] https://www.ncbi.nlm.nih.gov/pmc/articles/ PMC8470444/pdf

other antioxidant pigments.

The world of phytonutrients is vast and complex, with still much to be discovered. There are around 200,000 edible plants, each containing their own set of phytochemicals. Humans consume less than 300 of these plants.[19] Imagine the untapped potential! By eating a varied diet rich in colorful fruits, vegetables, whole grains, teas, spices, nuts, and seeds we can enjoy the wide range of phytonutrients. Many of these will have specific therapeutic benefits that can support us on our mental health journey.

---

[19] https://www.weforum.org/agenda/2016/01/why-do-we-consume-only-a-tiny-fraction-of-the-world-s-edible-plants/

Fermented Foods & Probiotics

Fermented foods are becoming increasingly popular due to their potential to support our gut microbiome. Fermentation is a process of converting carbohydrates into alcohol or acid, which helps to preserve food and create unique flavors. By consuming fermented foods, individuals can gain beneficial bacteria and enzymes that can help promote a balanced microbiome.

As we've discussed, the gut microbiome is a diverse population of bacteria, fungi, and viruses that live in our guts and play an essential role in our health. A well-tuned microbiome helps to regulate digestion, reduce inflammation, synthesize neurotransmitters, and enhance the immune system.

Fermented foods, such as kefir, yogurt, sauerkraut, kimchi, pickles, miso, and kombucha, contain beneficial bacteria that can help balance our gut microbiome. The lactic acid bacteria (LAB) found in fermented foods helps to break down carbohydrates, providing energy for the gut microbiome and preventing the growth of harmful bacteria. These fermented foods help restore beneficial gut bacteria and create an environment favorable for digestion and absorption of food. Additionally, the sour flavor of fermented foods encourages the production of saliva, which helps to break down food and promote digestion.

When it comes to mental health, research has begun to identify particular strains of bacteria that may significantly influence symptoms of anxiety and depression. For example, certain strains of Lactobacillus (found in most of the foods mentioned above) help produce neurotransmitters like GABA, which can influence mood and anxiety levels.

With the much-deserved hype around fermented food, we also hear a lot of praise for probiotics. Often, anything fermented is called a probiotic, but this is a misuse of the term. Probiotics are live microorganisms formulated and scientifically tested for specific therapeutic benefits. Fermented foods also contain beneficial bacteria, though present in smaller amounts. And, unlike a true probiotic, they cannot be said to confer a specific benefit to the host based on scientific evidence. But don't take this to mean fermented foods are inferior. In many cases, probiotics are unnecessary, and fermented foods consumed regularly will be enough to bring a steady supply of new critters to the microbial party. Two to six servings of fermented foods a day can work wonders!

Fermented foods play a major role in nurturing a healthy gut microbiome, which is essential for optimal mental health. A balanced gut promotes the production of key neurotransmitters like serotonin and dopamine, reduces inflammation, and enhances the gut-brain connection. While incorporating fermented foods can bolster beneficial gut bacteria, individuals with digestive disorders might require probiotics. If considering probiotics, you may benefit from consulting a doctor or nutritionist to determine the right type and dosage for your needs.

Adaptogens

Adaptogens are a fascinating group of herbs and mushrooms that uniquely support the body in navigating the challenges of physical, emotional, and environmental stress. Moreover, they're believed to sharpen mental clarity, energize the body, and enhance overall well-being.

So, how do adaptogens do all this? They help the body maintain balance during stressful times by regulating the HPA axis, a central pathway in stress regulation. This axis controls the body's stress response, including the release of cortisol, a key stress hormone.

Adaptogens can fine-tune cortisol levels, ensuring they're balanced for the body's needs.
Among the adaptogens studied for their impact on mental health, Rhodiola Siberian ginseng and Schisandra chinensis stand out. But others are worth mentioning as well. Here's a look at some of the more common adaptogens and their potential mental health benefits:

- **Ashwagandha**: Known for reducing anxiety and depression.

- **Ginseng**: Both American and Asian ginseng are used to boost energy, improve concentration, enhance physical stamina, and support overall well-being.

- **Rhodiola**: Aids in reducing fatigue, depression, and pain. It may enhance mental performance. Note: Rhodiola should not be taken daily as tolerance can be developed over time.

- **Astragalus root**: Thought to protect against stress and aging.

- **Siberian ginseng**: Often used to help adapt to physical and mental stress, reduce fatigue, and enhance immune function. Some studies show that it may enhance cognitive function and mood. It may also be beneficial for those experiencing chronic fatigue or mental exhaustion.

- **Holy basil (tulsi)**: Promotes relaxation and can help to relieve stress and anxiety.

- **Schisandra chinensis** (Chinese Magnolia Vine or Five-Flavor Berry): Known for its potential benefits in stress adaptation, as it may balance the nervous system and support adrenal function. It could also enhance cognitive functions like mental clarity, focus, and alertness, especially during stress or fatigue. Some studies have hinted at possible antidepressant effects, but more research is needed. Additionally, Schisandra might aid in improving sleep quality and addressing insomnia, though studies in this area are also limited.

- **Maca root powder**: Believed to uplift mood and reduce symptoms of depression and anxiety. It's also linked to improved cognitive function and memory.

There are a few mushrooms like reishi, chaga, and cordyceps, that are considered adaptogens as well but we will look at these in the next section.

The effectiveness of adaptogens in reducing stress and anxiety, improving mental focus, and boosting energy is supported by research, but further studies are needed to fully grasp their potential benefits for mental health.

Adaptogens offer a natural way to support the body's resilience to stress and enhance mental well-being. While promising, the field continues to evolve. It is recommended to first focus on a varied and balanced diet rich in plants, but you might try adding a few of these adaptogens to target specific enhancements.

Fungi

Mushrooms are a great way to add unique flavors and enhanced nutrition to your diet. They are low in calories, cholesterol-free, and can help boost your immune system. Current research is also finding that mushrooms can help reduce anxiety, depression, and sleep issues while also improving cognitive function and sex drive. There are even studies exploring how psychedelic mushrooms can be used to treat addiction and help us face death with less anxiety. That's a lot of support from our fungi friends!

Mushrooms are primarily composed of carbohydrates with small amounts of protein. They are also high in selenium and potassium. Though many antioxidants are found in plants, ergothioneine is only found in mushrooms. Mushrooms also contain certain types of prebiotic fiber, like beta-glucans, that can help improve digestive health.

Mushrooms are a great source of B vitamins such as B1, B2, B3, B5, and B9. They are also the only plant source of vitamin D. Much like our skin, mushrooms also create and store vitamin D after exposure to sunlight or other UV light sources.

Psilocybin is the psychoactive compound in "magic mushrooms." It is currently being studied as a possible treatment for various mental health issues, such as depression, anxiety, and obsessive-compulsive disorder. Other studies are exploring it as a potential aid for end-of-life care and as a potential tool for enhancing spiritual experiences. Additionally, researchers are investigating how psilocybin can be used in the treatment of alcoholism and smoking cessation.

Currently, psilocybin is a Schedule I illicit substance under the Controlled Substances Act in the USA. However, there are some exceptions. For example, Oregon has legalized psilocybin for therapeutic usage. In Colorado, Denver and Colorado Springs have decriminalized personal growing, use, and sharing of psilocybin and psilocin for adults. In 2022, Colorado legalized psilocybin and psilocin for use in therapeutic settings, paving the way for "healing centers" where adults 21 years old and up can use the substances under the supervision of licensed professionals. In some countries, such as Portugal and the Netherlands, psilocybin use is not criminalized.

I realize that not everyone will wait for their local government to follow the lead of some of these states and countries that are more progressive in their approach. Though we don't condone breaking the law, in the event that you plan on eating psychedelic mushrooms outside the places mentioned above, here are some harm reduction steps to consider:

1. Start with a low dose and gradually increase the dose over subsequent experiences.

2. Have a sober sitter present during your experience.

3. Set an intention for the experience and focus on that intention throughout.

4. Have a comfortable and secure environment.

5. Avoid taking psychedelics if you are not feeling well, either physically or mentally.

6. Avoid combining psychedelics with other drugs or alcohol.

7. Listen to your body and respect its signals.

8. Be aware of the possibility of having a difficult experience and plan for it. With support and integration, these "bad trips" can turn out to be extremely helpful and even transformative.

9. Integrate the experience afterward by writing or talking about it.

10. Consider joining a psychedelic support circle or organization to connect with a community of people who are also exploring psychedelics.

If eating mushrooms for a psychedelic journey is not your thing, there are many other options for experiencing the healing properties of mushrooms...

Here are some of my favorite mushrooms for mental health and wellness:

- **Chaga, cordyceps, reishi, and maitake mushrooms** are all adaptogens. Chaga and maitake mushrooms also have anti-inflammatory properties, which can help reduce inflammation and oxidation. Cordyceps have been used traditionally to manage exhaustion and fatigue. Chaga powder can be used in coffee or other hot beverages to stimulate creativity. Reishi mushrooms can help in relaxation and deeper sleep as they are a powerful tool for calming the mind and easing anxiety.

- **Turkey tail mushrooms** have antioxidant, antibacterial, and antiviral activity, helping to keep the body healthy and manage anxiety.

- **Porcini mushrooms** provide some protein and are rich in vitamins and minerals, including iron, vitamin A, and vitamin C. The amino acids they provide help to produce neurotransmitters that can reduce symptoms of depression and anxiety.

- **Crimini mushrooms** are also a great source of vitamins and minerals, including vitamins B2, B3, and B5, which fuel the brain.

- **Oyster mushrooms** contain an active compound called benzaldehyde, which has potent antibacterial and anti-inflammatory properties. This makes them great for people with chronic anxiety.

- **Lions mane mushrooms** have the remarkable ability to stimulate the production of nerve growth factor (NGF), which may promote the growth of new brain cells and cells in the gut, potentially enhancing cognitive function and supporting gut health.

- **Shiitake mushrooms** are rich in B vitamins, copper, selenium, and potassium. They are also a great source of dietary fiber and contain important compounds like beta-glucans which can help reduce stress and anxiety. Additionally, the antioxidants like ergothioneine in shiitake mushrooms may help protect against oxidative stress, which can be helpful with symptoms of anxiety and depression.

You can add mushroom tincture or powders to meals, mocktails, hot drinks, and smoothies. Introduce them one by one and find out which one makes a difference and how. Most are subtle. Cordyceps are not—you may feel like running a marathon on them!

Before taking adaptogens and medicinal mushrooms, consulting with herbalists, naturopaths, or other integrative healthcare practitioners can be helpful. These professionals are trained in the therapeutic use of botanicals and can provide personalized recommendations based on an individual's unique health needs, lifestyle, and medical history. They can help identify the most appropriate herbs or mushrooms for specific health goals, determine the correct dosages, and ensure that the chosen supplements do not interact negatively with any medications or other supplements being taken. By seeking guidance from experts in herbal medicine, individuals can safely and effectively incorporate adaptogens and medicinal mushrooms into their wellness routines, maximizing potential benefits while minimizing risks.

So, if you're looking for additional natural remedies to improve your overall mental health, consuming one of the many mushroom varieties available could be a healthy (and possibly transformative) option.

In this chapter, we've explored the systems and components that influence our mental health. The next chapter will introduce foundational principles for effecting change, enabling us to make informed choices that optimize these resources for peak mental and emotional well-being. By integrating this knowledge with practical strategies, you'll be equipped to effectively biohack your mood.

Strategy for Change

Goals & Visualizations

What if we start with the ending? Where do you imagine yourself if successful? Can you see it? Taste it? One of the questions therapists often ask when trying to help people change is "If you woke up one morning and your life felt different in a positive way, what would you notice had changed?" In Motivational Interviewing (an evidenced-based therapy focused on the stages of change), this is called the miracle question. The question can help us anchor to a future goal. If you can see what you want to be different, you can start working backward to build the steps needed to get there. Thoreau said, "If you've built your castles in the air, that is where they should be; now build the foundation."

When it comes to biohacking your mood with plant-based food, where do you hope this will lead you? I'm guessing you hope to feel happier, calmer, more focused, well-rested, and/or sexier. If any of these resonate with you, picture yourself feeling this way.

One theory proposes that to change, we must have an experience. Since therapy is about connecting us with how we feel, in order to feel different, we must experience our emotions. This is why "How does that make you feel" is a stereotypical therapist response. The hope is it will draw us out of our heads into our hearts to have a present-moment experience with an emotion.

But how do we experience a new behavior when part of the problem is that we are stuck in old patterns that deny the experience of this behavior? Enter the magic of the brain and the little trick of visualization. If we visualize something in our mind vividly enough, our brain can perceive the experience as genuine. How this translates: we create new neural pathways, making it easier to perform the task we have visualized ourselves completing successfully. It's like muscle memory, but we don't have to lift a finger. But how do we make the mental scene seem real? This is where we have to use our bodies and all our senses.

Here's an example:

Say you want to spend more time preparing one healthy meal a week. Each morning take 2-5 minutes sitting quietly with your eyes closed. (Some people are more able to actually picture the scene in their minds. Others may struggle to see the details clearly. Either way, just using your imagination can achieve what we are trying to do here.)

Okay, imagine yourself walking into your kitchen, opening the fridge, grabbing the veggies out of the crisper. Notice the temperature of the room and the subtle chill coming from the fridge. Feel the textures as you lift the veggies and place them on the counter. See all the ingredients laid out. Notice how you feel seeing the colors. See yourself setting up your cutting board and getting your favorite knife. Feel the weight of the handle. As you begin prepping the ingredients, hear the sound of the knife cutting through the vegetable and knocking against the chopping block. Imagine picking up a piece of the chopped veggies and tasting it. Now, start the cooking process: pan on the stove, a bit of oil heated, drop in your first ingredient, hear the sizzle, and smell the first aromas.

You get the picture. Now create one of your own. Vividly walk yourself through a mental movie of you succeeding at a one of your plant-based goals, and make sure to bring all five senses along for the experience.

Mindfulness

Our brain is designed for efficiency. It rewards us with dopamine for recognizing and adhering to patterns. Over time, as we repeatedly engage in specific behaviors, our brain strengthens certain neural pathways, making these behaviors almost automatic. While beneficial in many scenarios, this efficiency can sometimes lead us down paths of habit that aren't in our best interest. The more entrenched these habits become, the more challenging it is to deviate from them, as doing so requires more cognitive effort.

Mindfulness offers a way to break these automatic patterns. By cultivating awareness, we can observe our behaviors as they unfold, identifying opportunities to make different choices. The key is to catch ourselves early in the process.

For instance, if you have a routine of unwinding with a bag of Doritos in front of the television after work, disrupting this pattern, once you're already settled into your easy chair, might feel quite challenging. However, by introducing a mindful pause as soon as you step into your home—perhaps while taking off your shoes—you can consciously decide to head to the kitchen to prepare a healthy snack instead. While this redirection might still require effort, it's made easier by catching the habit at its onset.

To aid this transition, many find it helpful to pair their mindful pause with a deep breath. This simple act can serve as a reset, activating the parasympathetic nervous system and facilitating a more relaxed state. This relaxation can be especially beneficial when trying to break a pattern the brain is resistant to change.

Now, let's tie this into our relationship with food. By being present and attentive to our eating habits, we can discern how different foods influence our mood and overall well-being. This awareness can lead to more informed choices, fostering a healthier relationship with our meals. For instance, if we notice a pattern of feeling sluggish after consuming certain foods, mindfulness can help us recognize this connection and choose alternatives that better support our energy and mood. The next time we have an urge for that unhelpful food, we can pause, take a breath, divert our attention to a healthier option, and notice how we feel after eating it instead.

Mindfulness provides a framework for understanding and changing our habits, including food-related ones. By grounding ourselves in the present and observing our patterns without judgment, we can make choices that better align with our well-being goals.

Behavioral Modification

So, you have chosen a goal and the easiest first step you can imagine taking toward that goal. You've visualized yourself carrying out the steps to complete your goal. You are paying more attention to your automatic habits and considering where to insert a mindful pause so you can redirect toward the new action. These are the major components of modifying our behavior. But how do you make the behavior stick in the long term?

This is where behavioral science comes in. Remember old Pavlov and his salivating dog? It's all about associations. The dog learns that a bell means dinner is served. Once this neural pattern is set in the brain, even when dinner is removed from the equation, the dog will still slobber all over himself at the sound of a bell. How is this useful to us as we set out on the adventure of eating more plants?

We, too, have to hard wire in the new habit. We can take a couple of cues from the behaviorists. First, repetition is key. And it becomes infinitely easier to repeat something if it follows on from a pattern already being repeated without thought. Say, each morning, you have your coffee after getting out of bed.

This can be an anchor that you can pair with the new healthy habit. Maybe you want to start taking omega-3 algae supplements daily. With all the hustle and bustle of prepping breakfast, you keep forgetting to follow the meal with your algae pill. A possible solution is to set up an "if-then" scenario. You can plant a mental seed by telling yourself: *If* I have my morning coffee, *then* I will set my algae pill next to my breakfast items after pouring my cup of coffee.

Habits stick best when they become an integral part of your established routine. So, having them tag along with parts of the routine already set in stone allows us to bring them into the rhythm. And we know this rhythm works because it allows us to spend less mental energy making decisions. Whatever new plant-based goal you have, try anchoring it to something you're already doing, and try to have it occur around the same time each day.

There is no hard evidence about how long it takes our brains to lay down the tracks that establish a new habit—where it feels like less of a conscious choice and more like a simple automation—but the general rule is 60-90 days. You don't have to engage in the behavior every day for this length of time, but there are a couple of guidelines that can help: if you miss a day, no big deal; if you miss two days, put all your effort into figuring out how you'll get back on track the next day; if you miss three days, the habit formation process is going to feel like you are starting back at the beginning.

Once you get on a roll, it can be inspiring to see the days add up. Remember the gold star our teacher would stick on our chart for each day we behaved? The same concept works here. Getting a visual of our success feels good. There are lots of great habit-tracking apps that do this. Link days together and notice the positive feeling that grows the longer it gets.

It can also help to consider what motivates us. Why do you want to make this change? What about eating plants to improve your mental and emotional states inspires you? Basically, what is *your* why? Friedrich Nietzsche said, "He who has a why to live can bear almost any how." This speaks to the importance of purpose and meaning in life, suggesting that when we have a strong reason or purpose, a 'why,' we can endure and overcome challenges and hardships, the 'how.' This can be the foundation from which we build the structured steps toward what we want to put in place for our future. I won't give examples here, as genuine inspiration needs to come from within you; the phrasing must cause you to feel motivated. So, for you, why change? Why do you want things to be different?

Finally, there's a concept in bird watching (or "birding" if you're in the "club") called the spark bird. The spark bird is the bird that ignites the passion. Often, it catches you off guard. There is a randomness to the occurrence. What gets us hooked on the various things we are captivated by? Often, there's a moment, and something in that moment strikes us.

Thinking back to my evolving relationship with plant-based food, I am curious about what (beyond wanting to be a hippie) initially grabbed my attention. What made it such a priority in my life that, like the birders, it didn't matter if others (in this case, my meat-loving family—I grew up on a farm, where my pet pig found its way to my dinner plate) thought it was a strange thing to get up to? I'd probably say it had something to do with tempeh, specifically tempeh burgers. With this discovery, I realized it didn't feel like I was giving up much when turning my back on beef patties.

On your plant-based eating journey, stay on the lookout for your "spark plant." What plant food tips the balance for you, and makes changing your eating habits more effortless because you have "caught the bug?"

So, we've put together the different components that can help you move toward your end goal. But there is one extra step, that for many people, is the thing that ignites the fire of motivation: the reward. For some people, achievement is the reward. But most of us want a bit more than that. We want to feel celebrated for our accomplishments. So celebrate. Buy yourself something you will look forward to. Or take yourself out to a nice plant-based restaurant. If new toys are your thing, there are plenty of kitchen appliances that can take your plant-based food adventure to another level. I recently bought a Ninja air fryer: game changer.

Incorporating these strategies and understanding the psychology behind habit formation can set you on a path to long-term success in achieving your plant-based goals. By embracing behavioral science principles and aligning new habits with existing routines, you can anchor your desired changes into your daily life. Remember, the journey towards a healthier and more plant-based lifestyle isn't just about achieving a goal; it's about relishing the transformation itself. In the upcoming section, we'll delve into the joys of embracing the process and finding delight in each step of your journey towards a more plant-centered way of living.

Enjoy the Process

Though we resist change (for the reason already mentioned: our brains are a bit lazy and want to conserve energy by sticking with the old familiar route), the process can be enjoyable if we intend to make it that way. Though wading through a mound of food blogs and the never-ending slew of Instagram food porn to come up with a weekly menu can be daunting at first, once we get a sense of what we like, what foods are easy to locate in our local market, and have established some basic kitchen routines, there is an element of playfulness (and even adventure) found in eating to support our mental health.

As you gain confidence in crafting your weekly menu, figure out what foods work well together to offer the proper nutrients that help you feel better, and find your rhythm in the kitchen, you may be surprised at how fun and rewarding the process can be.

Here are a few ideas that can enhance the experience:

- Tell friends about your goal and talk about what you are learning. Bonus points if in the conversation, you are able to talk about your own mental health journey and help diminish some of the stereotypes around this topic.

- Post pictures of your latest meal creation on Facebook or Instagram.

- Find a local farmers market and make it a goal to locate one new plant you've never cooked with.

- Purchase and use a new kitchen tool like a mandolin, spiralizer, or air fryer to level up your game.

- Fall in love with nutritional yeast ('nooch') and all the "cheesy" creations you can concoct with it.

- Try making your own meat substitutes like cauliflower meatballs, jackfruit-pulled "pork," or seitan.

- Learn how to ferment (you can do this with just about any plant food) and offer this gift as a "thank you" to your wonderful gut microbiota.

- Try to eat a 3-course meal without a white or beige thing on your plate.

- Track your micronutrient intake and mood over the course of a month or two as an experiment (check out healthymoods.org for tools to help you do just that).

- Explore local plant-based restaurants, find your favorite dish, and try to create your own version of it at home.

- Start using more fresh herbs both to enhance the nutrient density in your meals but also as a garnish to make the plate presentation more lively.

- Learn the art of "reading" your poo for signs of good health or potential gut issues.

- Volunteer on a local farm. As an exchange, you'll often come away with a load of fresh produce and likely an item or two you don't usually buy but that can help you add a new dish to your menu.

- Make your own plant-based milk or cheese.

- Make cooking an exercise in mindfulness. The process can be an act of self-care and, if done in this fashion, can be just the opposite of another stressful task to add to a busy schedule.

- See if you can include 30 different plant foods in your weekly menu.

- Take a course on plating or plant-based cooking to develop your culinary skills further. The Plant Academy in the UK offers some great online and in-person options.

- Track your fiber intake and see if you can consistently get around 50g/day.

- Challenge yourself to get 2-6 servings of

fermented foods a day.

- Treat yourself to a new cookbook. *Mind Food* by Lauren Lovatt offers many top-notch recipes that are designed to support your mental health.

Learning anything new can be a drag if we only experience resistance to this new way of doing things. Again, the brain prefers old patterns, so forcing it to break out of the "old mindset" to create some new inroads will contain an element of struggle. But that struggle is compounded if we focus on just that aspect of the process. So, focus on a few elements that you enjoy. Bring the intention of openness and excitement into the journey. Notice how you develop new skills and more profound knowledge of the food-mood connection over time. And feel proud of yourself for taking the initiative to take better care of yourself through the way you eat.

Flow

Eating a plant-based diet can be a powerful tool for optimizing mental health. But it's not only about what you eat—it's also about how you prepare and consume your food. With so many options and the time and thought that goes into planning and preparation, it can seem like a lot of effort initially. I want to make the process as simple and enjoyable for you as possible. I want to help you find a way to streamline the process, maximizing the benefits of eating plants. In short, I want to help you *flow* as you engage in this food-mood dance, gracefully maneuvering through your kitchen as you wield various instruments and whip up some exquisite and nutritious meals that help you feel your best.

Flow is all about patterns. When we have established habits or daily rituals that become so automatic that we don't have to stop to think about the next step, we just "flow." Again, as I've been promoting throughout this book, the brain, as wonderful as it is, can't get in our way. We overthink things. We rely on the cognitive process, developing its capacities, at the expense of other essential aspects immediately available to us: emotions, our bodies (somatic experiences), and unconscious processes.

Though this is an oversimplification—the actual

workings of the brain are much more complex and involve interactions between various regions—the left brain hemisphere is more involved with logic and reasoning, while the right hemisphere allows for creativity and intuition. Flow uses both hemispheres toward a more effortless state.

To help you get into the flow of things with your plant-based diet, the next chapter will offer some tips and tricks that you can implement to optimize your mental and emotional health. You have utilized your left brain to digest and think about how plant foods and various systems work together to support how you feel. Now, we will look at specific actions you can take that will activate these systems to maximize their effectiveness. Take these steps often enough, listen to how your body responds, and begin to trust your gut about which actions to stick with and which to discard, and you will be cultivating right-brain activities that will improve your ability to flow throughout the process.

By integrating some of these action steps into your cooking and eating routine, you won't have to stop and think about the hows and whys. Instead, you can establish new habitual patterns that allow you to move through your kitchen and connect with your food with little effort. The foods you create will energize your gut army, nourish your brain, and enhance neurotransmitter production. The result? You can feel less stressed, more focused, happier, and perhaps even a little sexier.

In the next chapter, we'll break these tips and tricks into categories based on what you've learned so far.

But first, we'll look at ways to optimize your kitchen setup for efficiency.

Tips & Tricks

Kitchen Setup

In the world of culinary arts, we're often inundated with advertisements and recommendations for a myriad of kitchen gadgets, leading us to believe we need a vast array of tools to cook effectively. However, the truth is, a well-equipped kitchen can be quite minimalistic. At the core, the essentials include:

- Two pots (medium and large)
- One frying pan
- Grater box
- Stainless steel peeler
- Three knives (paring, serrated, and chopping)
- Wooden chopping block
- Baking tray
- Roasting tray
- Scale
- Sieve
- Casserole dish

While these tools form the foundation of a functional kitchen, there are a few non-essential items that, based on my experience, can elevate your cooking game: an air fryer, which can save time as well as money (being more energy-efficient than an oven); a mini-blender like the Nutribullet, perfect for whipping up smoothies, cashew creams, or grinding seeds; and a food processor, which is a game-changer for concocting hummus, salsa, energy balls and more.

An efficient kitchen focuses on maximizing functionality while minimizing clutter. Here are some tips to achieve such a setup:

Prioritize: Think about your cooking habits. If you bake a lot, invest in good baking tools. If you're more into stovetop cooking, prioritize quality pots and pans.

Limit Single-Use Gadgets: Avoid tools that serve only one purpose unless you use them very frequently. For example, an avocado slicer might be unnecessary if a knife does the job just as well. Believe me, I feel for this one; an avocado slicer is rarely used.

Declutter Regularly: Periodically go through your kitchen items and donate or discard tools and appliances you haven't used in the past year.

Quality Over Quantity: Instead of having multiple versions of the same tool, invest in one high-quality version that will last longer and perform better.

Limit Dishware: You don't need a full set of 12 plates, bowls, and glasses unless you frequently host large gatherings. Keep enough for your household plus a few extras for guests.

Regular Maintenance: Take care of your tools. Regularly sharpen knives, season cast iron pans, and clean appliances. This extends their life and reduces the need for replacements.

Organized Storage: Use drawer dividers, pot racks, and clear storage containers (empty jars from items you've purchased are great for this!) to keep everything organized. Being able to easily see and access what you have prevents unnecessary purchases.

Open Shelving: This not only saves space but also forces you to keep only what you need and use regularly, as everything is in plain sight.

Maximize Vertical Space: Use wall-mounted racks for utensils, pots, and pans. This keeps them easily accessible and saves drawer and cabinet space.

Streamlined Pantry: Keep a basic set of versatile ingredients on hand. This reduces the need for last-minute shopping trips and helps in creating a variety of dishes with a limited pantry.

Digital Cookbooks: Instead of physical cookbooks, consider using digital versions or apps. They take up no physical space and are easily searchable.

Fridge Temp: Different plant-based foods have different optimal storage temperatures. Keeping them at the right temperature can significantly extend their shelf life. Ensure that your fridge is set to the right temperature (typically between 35°F and 38°F or 1.7°C to 3.3°C).

Hydroponic cultivation: Growing herbs in water is a great way to have fresh herbs all year round without the need for soil. Basil, mint, oregano, rosemary, sage, and chive are some herbs that thrive when grown this way.

In essence, the goal of a minimalist kitchen is to create a functional, efficient space that makes cooking enjoyable and stress-free. By focusing on essentials and organizing effectively, you can reduce clutter, save money, and make your culinary endeavors more enjoyable.

Saving Time & Money

Cooking is as much an art as it is a science. While creativity plays a role in crafting delicious dishes, efficiency in preparation and the cooking process ensures that meals are not only tasty but also timely. Mastering a few key techniques can significantly streamline your kitchen endeavors, making the experience more enjoyable and less time-consuming.

Plan Ahead: If you know you'll be short on time, consider prepping the main ingredients, marinating proteins, or soaking grains and legumes the night before. This reduces active cooking time the next day.

Organize Your Workspace: Group ingredients and tools by the order you'll use them. This "assembly line" approach ensures you're not wasting time searching for what you need next.

Batch Cooking: Dedicate a day or a few hours in the week to cook meals or components of meals in large quantities. This approach is especially useful for those with busy schedules. Once cooked, these meals or components can be stored in the refrigerator or freezer and reheated throughout the week, saving time on daily meal prep. If you know you'll be using certain ingredients multiple times during the week (like chopped onions or minced garlic), prep them in larger quantities and store in the fridge. This way, you have them ready to go for multiple meals. I often take Sunday afternoon to make batches of salsa, hummus, granola, tamari almonds, cashew cream, and kombucha.

Bench scrapers: Also known as "dough scrapers," these flat, rectangular tools can be used in baking to manipulate and cut dough, but they are also handy in general cooking for transferring chopped ingredients from the cutting board to a pan or bowl.

Mise en Place: This French term translates to "everything in its place." It involves preparing and organizing ingredients before the actual cooking begins. Using small bowls, like ramekins, to hold pre-measured ingredients can be a game-changer. Not only does it ensure that everything is at hand when needed, but it also allows chefs to focus solely on the cooking process, leading to a more efficient and enjoyable experience.

Sharp Knives: A sharp knife not only makes cutting easier but also safer. It reduces the effort required and ensures clean, precise cuts. Regularly sharpen your knives to maintain their edge.

One-Pot Meals: Dishes like stews, casseroles, and stir-fries allow you to cook multiple ingredients together in one pot or pan. This not only saves time but also reduces the number of dishes to clean.

Use a Timer: Instead of constantly checking on your food, set a timer. This allows you to focus on other tasks or prep work without the risk of overcooking. You don't need to purchase a kitchen timer for this; simply use your phones timer app.

Clean as You Go: Instead of leaving all the cleaning until after cooking, try to wash tools and dishes as you use them. This reduces the post-cooking cleanup and keeps your workspace tidy.

Steam Vegetables Over Grains: Towards the end of cooking grains like rice or quinoa, place a steamer basket of vegetables on top. This allows you to steam the vegetables for about 5 minutes, making the most of the heat and saving time.

Use Technology: There are numerous apps and tools that can help with meal planning, grocery lists, and recipe organization. Leveraging these can save time in planning and shopping.

By incorporating these techniques into your kitchen routine, you'll find that cooking becomes less of a chore and more of a delightful activity, where efficiency and flavor go hand in hand.

Reducing Waste

In the journey towards sustainability, the kitchen plays a pivotal role. As more individuals transition to plant-based diets, the importance of minimizing waste becomes even more pronounced. A plant-based kitchen, with its array of fruits, vegetables, legumes, and grains, offers numerous opportunities to repurpose and reuse, ensuring that every part of the produce is utilized to its fullest. From using leftover pulp from juicing to finding creative ways to store perishables, every step taken towards reducing waste not only benefits the environment but also enhances the nutritional value and flavor of our meals. Moreover, by maximizing the use of every ingredient, we can significantly reduce food costs, making plant-based eating both eco-friendly and budget-friendly. Here are a few tips that can help:

Save the Gold

Explanation: The liquid that chickpeas come in is called aquafaba or liquid gold. It is a good source of plant-based protein, fiber, and some micronutrients like iron and potassium. Aquafaba is a versatile vegan substitute for eggs, especially in baking and cooking.

Action Step: Whip it to mimic egg whites in dishes like meringues and vegan mayonnaise. Its sticky nature makes it an effective binder for recipes such as veggie burgers. Additionally, its unique properties allow it to be used in a variety of vegan desserts, from ice cream to marshmallows. When sweetened, it can be transformed into a light vegan whipped cream, and it can also enhance the texture of drinks, adding creaminess to smoothies and frothiness to cocktails.

Store Foods Separately

Explanation: Some fruits and vegetables release ethylene gas, which can cause other produce to ripen and spoil faster.

Action Step: Keep ethylene-producing foods (like apples and bananas) away from ethylene-sensitive foods (like leafy greens and berries). Though, you can also use this trick to ripen fruits like avocado faster: simply stick the avocado in a paper bag with a banana and it should ripen in one to three days.

Spring Onions/Asparagus in Water

Explanation: Just like cut flowers, these veggies can absorb water from their cut ends, keeping them fresh.

Action Step: Trim the ends, place them upright in a glass with an inch of water, and cover the tops with a plastic bag. Store on the counter.

Herbs in Damp Paper Towels

Explanation: Herbs can dry out quickly in the fridge. Keeping them in a damp environment helps retain their moisture.

Action Step: Wrap herbs in a damp paper towel, place them in a plastic bag, and store in the fridge. If you have fresh herbs that you can't use up quickly, chop them and freeze them in ice cube trays with olive oil or water. This way, you have pre-portioned herbs ready to drop into dishes.

Cucumbers with Ventilation

Explanation: Cucumbers can get soggy if they're in a sealed environment.

Action Step: Store them outside the fridge in a plastic bag with holes for airflow.

Mushrooms in Paper Bags

Explanation: Mushrooms can become slimy if stored in plastic. Paper absorbs excess moisture, keeping them dry.

Action Step: Store mushrooms in a paper bag in the fridge.

Avocado with Onion

Explanation: Onion emits sulfur gases that prevent the browning enzyme in avocados from working.

Action Step: Store a cut avocado with a chunk of onion in an airtight container.

Ginger in the Freezer

Explanation: Ginger can dry out or mold quickly at room temperature.

Action Step: Store whole ginger in the freezer. Grate or slice directly from frozen when needed.

Use Banana Peels

Explanation: Banana peels are rich in essential nutrients like vitamin C, vitamin B6, and potassium. They are also where the majority of a bananas fiber is found.

Action Step: Chop up and use in oatmeal, stir fies, smoothies, etc.

Date Seed Coffee

Explanation: Date seed coffee is not only a great caffeine-free alternative but also offers various health benefits. It's rich in antioxidants, and some studies suggest it may have anti-inflammatory properties.

Action Step: Spread seeds on a tray and dry either in the sun for several days or in an oven set to 150°F (65°C) for a few hours. Once dried, roast them at 325°F (165°C) for 20-30 minutes until they turn dark brown, ensuring you stir occasionally. Grind and brew using 2 tablespoons per cup. This can be brewed using methods like a French press, a standard coffee maker, or the drip method.

Don't Throw Out the Fiber

Explanation: When juicing fruits and vegetables, a significant amount of fiber is often left behind. Remember this is valuable food for your gut microbes!

Action Step: Instead of discarding this nutrient-rich pulp, incorporate it into oatmeal, breads, or muffins.

Utilize Broccoli Stems

Explanation: Broccoli stems are often discarded in favor of the florets, but they are just as nutritious and flavorful. They are packed with fiber, vitamin C, and calcium, making them a valuable part of the vegetable.

Action Step: Peel the tough outer layer of the stem and then slice, dice, or julienne the inner part. These can be added to stir-fries, salads, or soups. You can also blend them into smoothies or make a broccoli stem slaw as a crunchy side dish.

Carleigh over at Plantyou.com has a whole series on creative ways to use your food scraps, many of which will be included in her new cookbook, *Scrappy Cooking.*

Embracing a plant-based lifestyle not only champions environmental consciousness but also underscores the importance of maximizing every ingredient's potential. By adopting these practical tips, we can ensure that our culinary endeavors are not only flavorful and nutritious but also eco-friendly and cost-effective.

Gut Health Tips

With the increasing understanding of the gut's importance, it is important to seek ways to nourish and maintain a balanced gut microbiome. Incorporating a diverse range of foods that are rich in prebiotics, beneficial bacteria, and essential fibers is key. Here are some invaluable tips to supercharge your gut health and ensure it thrives:

Onion Options: Onions are a fantastic source of prebiotics, which feed the beneficial bacteria in your gut. But did you know that different types of onions contain different types of prebiotics? By using a variety of onions in your cooking—red, yellow, white, shallots, green onions—you're providing a diverse menu for your gut bacteria, promoting a healthier and more balanced gut microbiome.

Psyllium Husk Helper: Psyllium husk is a form of fiber that acts as a prebiotic, feeding your gut bacteria and promoting regular bowel movements. Try adding a teaspoon of psyllium husk to your morning smoothie, your oatmeal, or even your baking recipes for a gut-friendly fiber boost.

Miso Magic: Miso is a fermented soybean paste that's rich in beneficial bacteria that support gut health. While it's a staple in soups, try thinking outside the box. Add a spoonful of miso to your salad dressings, marinades, hummus, or even your oatmeal.

Sauerkraut Snacking: Sauerkraut isn't just for topping sausages. This fermented cabbage powerhouse of beneficial microbes. Try topping your salads, sandwiches, stir-fry, savory pancakes, or even pizza with it. You can also enjoy it straight from the jar as a gut-healthy snack. Remember to drink the juice!

Tempeh Transformation: Tempeh is a fermented soy product that's packed with beneficial bacteria. But don't just slice and fry it. Crumble it up and use it as a ground meat substitute in your favorite recipes for a gut-friendly twist.

Kombucha Kick: Kombucha is a tea that's fermented by a symbiotic community of microbes. While it's delicious on its own, try using it as a mixer in your favorite cocktails or mocktails for a gut-boosting beverage.

Garlic Goodness: Garlic is a potent prebiotic, feeding the beneficial bacteria in your gut. To maximize its gut health benefits, crush your garlic and let it sit for a few minutes before cooking. This allows it to produce allicin, a compound with powerful health benefits.

Banana Boost: Bananas, particularly underripe ones, are rich in resistant starch, a type of fiber that acts as a prebiotic. In many cultures, underripe bananas and plantains are cooked in savory dishes. They can be boiled, fried, or baked. They can also be thinly sliced and dehydrated to make banana chips.

Apple Cider Advantage: Apple cider vinegar can help promote a healthy gut by encouraging the growth of beneficial bacteria. Try adding a splash to your salads, marinades, or even your morning glass of water.

Whole Grain Gain: Whole grains are rich in fiber, which is essential for a healthy gut. But don't just stick to whole wheat. Experiment with less common whole grains like spelt, kamut, or teff for a diverse fiber intake that your gut bacteria will love.

Apple Core Concept: Surprisingly, a significant portion of an apple's beneficial bacteria is found in its core. While many people discard the core, consuming it can provide a boost to your gut's microbial diversity. And, yes, though the seeds contain small amounts of compounds that can be harmful in large quantities, they are generally safe to eat.

Papaya Power: Papayas are not only delicious but also packed with enzymes like papain that aid digestion. This tropical fruit can help break down proteins in your gut, promoting a smoother digestive process and supporting gut health.

Dirt Won't Hurt: Out of habit or fear of dirt, we often peel off the skin on root vegetables, tossing away a valuable part of the plant. Plus, the bit of dirt it may contain could have microbes that can be good for your gut. Consider leaving the skin on vegetables like carrots and beets to benefit from the extra fiber, nutrients, and beneficial bacteria. One thing to consider: if the vegetable is not organic, peeling them may help reduce exposure to any pesticides.

Incorporating these foods and practices into diet can significantly enhance your gut health, leading to improved digestion, increased energy, and even a better mood. Remember, a happy gut often translates to a happier, healthier you.

Anti-Inflammation Tips

Antioxidants are nature's defense mechanism, helping to neutralize free radicals in our bodies. These free radicals can cause oxidative stress, which has been linked to a host of health issues. While supplements are available, antioxidants work their best when consumed naturally in food. Here are some tips to maximize the benefits of these powerful compounds in your daily diet.

The Darker the Better: Generally, the darker the color of a plant food, the higher its antioxidant content will be. So, choosing black beans over white beans or red grapes over green is a better option if trying to boost your antioxidant intake.

Pair Turmeric with Pepper: Turmeric contains curcumin, a compound with potent anti-inflammatory and antioxidant benefits. However, curcumin's absorption is limited in our body. To enhance its uptake, pair it with black pepper. Piperine, found in black pepper, can boost curcumin absorption by up to

2,000%[20]. So, when using turmeric, always add a pinch of black pepper to unlock its full potential.

Opt for Dark Chocolate: Dark chocolate, especially with 70% cocoa or more, is a treasure trove of flavonoids, caffeine, and theobromine, which can enhance brain function. To reap its benefits, indulge in one or two ounces daily.

Cook with Herbs: Herbs like rosemary, sage, and thyme are not just flavor enhancers. They come packed with anti-inflammatory and antioxidant properties beneficial for brain health. When using them, ensure they are not overcut or bruised to preserve their potency.

Spike Your Coffee: Elevate your morning brew with spices like cinnamon, ginger, and turmeric. These spices are known for their anti-inflammatory properties. Create a mix using 1 tsp ground turmeric, 1 tsp ground cinnamon, 1/2 tsp ground black pepper, and 1/2 tsp ground ginger. Add a 1/2 teaspoon to your coffee for a healthy twist.

Chomp Your Broccoli: Broccoli and other cruciferous vegetables like cauliflower and kale contain sulforaphane, a compound studied for its neuroprotective effects and antioxidant properties. Chewing or chopping these vegetables releases more of the beneficial compound. Cooking can reduce the levels of sulforaphane in vegetables, so lightly steaming or consuming is best if you want the full benefit. Adding mustard seed powder when cooking

---

[20] https://pubmed.ncbi.nlm.nih.gov/27111639/

cruciferous vegetables can boost sulforaphane levels further.

Tomatoes and Olive Oil: Combine the antioxidant power of tomatoes with the healthy fats of olive oil. The fats enhance the absorption of lycopene, a potent antioxidant in tomatoes.

Lemon Enhancement: Lemon can improve the absorption of catechins, powerful antioxidants found in green tea. Even adding a squeeze of lemon to a cup of green tea can make a difference.

Incorporate Cacao: Cacao is a rich source of antioxidants. Sprinkle cacao nibs on salads, blend them into smoothies, or even incorporate cacao into savory dishes like gravies.

Including some of these tips in your dietary habits can significantly enhance your antioxidant intake. Remember, a diet rich in plant-based foods like berries, beans, leafy greens, and the occasional chocolate ensures a steady supply of these beneficial compounds, helping shield your body from oxidative stress.

Tips for 30 Plants a Week

Diversifying our diet with a variety of plants is essential for optimal health. Aiming for 30 different plants a week might sound daunting, but with a few creative tweaks, it's an achievable goal. Here are some tips to effortlessly increase the number of plants in your diet and meet that target:

Broaden Your Horizons: If you usually buy one kind of bean, grain, or flour, next time you're at the store, pick up two or three alternative varieties to try.

Use Leafy Greens as Wraps: Swap out traditional bread or tortillas with romaine, collard, or Swiss chard leaves. These greens are rich in B vitamins, essential for brain health, and offer a fresh, crunchy alternative to processed grains.

Mix Leafy Greens in Sauces: Elevate your sauces by blending in greens like spinach, beet greens, or kale. For a twist on traditional pesto, use arugula (rocket), parsley, or spinach instead. This not only boosts the nutrient content but also adds a vibrant color to your dishes.

Sweeten Oats Naturally: Instead of using processed sugars, cook your oats with a blended mix of banana and a couple of dates. This natural sweetener is not only delicious but also adds to your plant count.

Sprinkle Sprouts on Granola: For an added crunch and a nutritional boost, sprinkle a handful of sprouts on your morning granola or yogurt bowl.

Diverse Dips: Experiment with different bases for your dips. Instead of just hummus with chickpeas, try making it with white beans. Or expand beyond hummus and try making dips from lentils, black beans, or even roasted beets. Each offers a unique flavor and adds to your weekly plant count.

Stir-fry Variety: When making stir-fries, throw in a variety of colorful veggies. Think beyond bell peppers and broccoli; add snap peas, bok choy, or even thinly sliced Brussels sprouts.

Herb Garnishes: Don't just use herbs for flavor; make them a prominent part of your dish. Garnish salads, soups, and even pasta with generous amounts of fresh herbs like cilantro, dill, or mint.

Seed Toppings: Seeds like chia, flax, and hemp can be sprinkled on almost anything—from salads to smoothies. They're a great way to add texture, nutrition, and increase your plant variety.

Frozen Veggies: Always keep a stash of frozen vegetables in your freezer. They're a quick and easy way to add more plants to your meals, especially when you're short on fresh produce.

Fruit Desserts: Instead of traditional desserts, opt for fruit-based ones. Make a fruit salad, bake an apple with cinnamon, or blend frozen berries with a splash of almond milk for a quick sorbet.

Incorporating a diverse range of plants into your diet not only provides a spectrum of nutrients but also supports a healthy gut microbiome. With these tips, reaching the goal of 30 plants a week becomes not just feasible but also an enjoyable culinary adventure.

Nutrient Tips

Incorporating a variety of nutrient-rich foods into your diet is essential for overall health. However, the way you prepare and combine these foods can significantly impact the nutrients you absorb. Here are some tips to maximize the nutritional benefits of your meals:

Cook Beans with Seaweed: Enhance the nutritional profile of your beans by adding seaweed. Seaweed is not only nutrient-dense but also helps soften beans and reduce their gas-producing properties.

Soak Your Grains and Legumes: Reduce phytic acid levels in grains and legumes by soaking them. This process enhances the absorption of essential minerals and makes them easier to digest. Soaking legumes and grains has also been shown to increase their GABA concentration.[21]

Use Nutritional Yeast: Boost your B-vitamin intake, especially B12, by sprinkling nutritional yeast on your dishes. It's a flavorful addition to popcorn, soups, and vegan cheese sauces.

Mind Your Iron Intake: To maximize iron

---

[21] https://www.ncbi.nlm.nih.gov/pmc/articles/PMC5986471/

absorption, avoid consuming coffee or tea an hour before or after eating iron-rich foods. Polyphenols in these beverages can inhibit iron absorption.

Opt for Frozen Produce: Frozen berries and greens often retain more nutrients than their fresh counterparts and are more cost-effective.

Boost Iron Absorption with Vitamin C: Consuming foods high in vitamin C with iron-rich plant foods can enhance the absorption of iron.

Maximize Nutrient Absorption from Seeds: The healthy fats in seeds can increase the absorption of protective nutrients in vegetables consumed in the same meal. For better nutrient absorption, consider grinding seeds, especially flaxseeds and chia seeds.

Unlock Garlic's Full Potential: Chopping or pressing garlic releases a compound called allicin, which has numerous health benefits. For optimal benefits, let chopped or pressed garlic sit for at least 5-10 minutes before consuming or cooking.

Pair Avocado with Kale: The healthy fats in avocado enhance the absorption of fat-soluble vitamins, like vitamin K, found in kale.

Give Your Seeds a Bath: Soaking seeds can enhance their digestibility and nutrient availability.

Sunbathe Your Mushrooms: Exposing mushrooms to sunlight can increase their vitamin D content. For maximum absorption, mushrooms should be exposed to UV light for at least an hour per day.

Being mindful of how you prepare and combine foods,

ensures that you're getting the most out of every bite. Remember, it's not just about what you eat, but also how you prepare and eat it.

Complete Protein Tips

Including complete proteins in a plant-based diet is essential for ensuring you get all the essential amino acids your body needs. While many animal sources naturally provide complete proteins, plant-based sources often need to be combined to achieve the same effect. Fortunately, there are several plant-based foods that are naturally complete proteins on their own (see the macronutrients section on proteins), and numerous delicious combinations that can help you achieve your protein goals. Here's some helpful combos to keep in mind:

Black Beans and Corn Tortillas: Combining a legume with a whole grain ensures a complete protein profile.

Brown Rice and Beans: A classic combination that provides all the essential amino acids.

Salad with Kidney Beans and Sunflower Seeds: Mixing a legume with seeds in your salad ensures you're getting a complete protein.

Whole Grain Bread and Nut Butter: A simple and delicious way to get a complete protein.

Quinoa and Lentils: Both delicious on their own, but when combined, they provide all the essential amino acids.

Hummus and Whole Grain Pita: A Middle Eastern favorite that's not only delicious but also a complete protein source.

Incorporating complete proteins into your diet is crucial, especially if you're following a plant-based or vegetarian lifestyle. By being mindful of your protein sources and ensuring you're combining foods effectively, you can easily meet your protein needs and enjoy a diverse and delicious diet.

Good Fat Tips

Healthy fats are not only beneficial for overall health but are crucial for brain health. Omega-3 fatty acids, in particular, play a vital role in cognitive function and mood regulation. While many associate these fats with fish, there are numerous plant-based sources that can help you meet your needs. Here are some tips to ensure you're getting an ample amount of these brain-boosting fats:

Creamy Tahini Pasta: Transform your pasta dishes by adding tahini to your tomato sauce. This creamy sesame seed paste not only enhances the flavor but also boosts the dish's omega-3 content.

Add Seeds to Your Diet: Seeds, especially flax, chia, and hemp, are powerhouses of omega-3s. You can incorporate them into various meals for added texture and nutrition. I use a six-seed mix (flax, chia, hemp, sesame, pumpkin, and sunflower) in oatmeal, smoothies, or yogurt most days.

Chia Seeds and Almond Milk: Pair chia seeds with almond milk for better absorption of their healthy fats.

Turmeric and Omega-3s: As you've probably noticed by now, turmeric is a rock-star in the world of plants that help with mental health. As already mentioned, there is a synergistic relationship between black pepper and turmeric. However, this combination not only boosts absorption but also aids in converting shorter-chain omega-3s, like those in chia seeds, to longer-chain omega-3s. Longer-chain omega-3s are particularly beneficial for brain health and other physiological functions.

Nut Butter Bliss: Create a creamy, omega-3 rich spread by making your own walnut butter. This nut butter can be a delightful addition to toast, smoothies, or even as a dip.

Algae Oil: Swap out your regular cooking oil with algae oil occasionally. It's a direct plant source of DHA and EPA, making it a fantastic alternative for those avoiding fish.

Purslane in Salads: This often-overlooked leafy green is a hidden gem in the world of omega-3s. Add it to your salads for a unique flavor and a dose of healthy fats.

Grind Your Seeds: Whole flaxseeds can pass through the digestive tract undigested, which means you might not gain all of their nutritional benefits. Grinding flaxseeds breaks them down, making it easier for your body to digest and absorb the nutrients, including their omega-3 fatty acid content. Chia seeds can be absorbed in both whole and ground forms, but grinding them might enhance the bioavailability of their nutrients as well.

Incorporating some of these tips into your eating routine can significantly enhance your intake of plant-based omega-3s. Remember, it's not just about adding these foods to your diet, but also about combining them effectively to maximize absorption. By prioritizing these healthy fats, you're taking a protective step towards our mental health.

Tips for Flavor

While plant-based ingredients are naturally flavorful, certain techniques and additions can elevate their taste to new heights. Here are some tips to help you achieve a rich and robust flavor in your vegan dishes:

Add Citrus Acid: A splash of citrus, whether it's lemon, lime, or orange, can instantly brighten up a dish and enhance its flavors.

Tomato Paste: Deepen the flavor of your sauces by adding a dollop of tomato paste. It adds a rich umami taste that complements various dishes.

Porcini Mushroom Powder: This concentrated mushroom powder is a secret weapon that also adds a burst of umami. A little goes a long way in soups, stews, and sauces.

Umami Broth Blend: Create a flavorful broth using dried mushrooms, salt, garlic powder, and optional kelp seaweed. This blend can be the base for various dishes, infusing them with a savory depth.

Use Kosher Salt: Opt for Diamond Crystal kosher salt when cooking. It's less salty than table salt, allowing for better control over seasoning. Reserve sea salt for finishing dishes or for recipes where its unique texture and flavor can shine, such as in desserts or raw dishes.

Fresh Herbs: Incorporate fresh herbs like basil, cilantro, or rosemary at the end of the cooking process. They add a burst of flavor and aroma that can transform a dish.

Curcumin: Derived from turmeric, curcumin not only offers health benefits but also imparts a warm, earthy flavor to dishes. Use it in curries, apple crisp, oatmeal, soups, or even smoothies for a flavor and health boost.

Roast Your Garlic: Instead of using raw garlic, try roasting it. Roasted garlic becomes sweet and creamy, adding a mellow and rich flavor to dishes.

Slow Cooked Onions: Taking the time to slowly caramelize onions can add a sweet, savory depth to dishes. They're perfect for sauces, stews, or even as a topping.

Pestle and Mortar: Grinding spices with a pestle and mortar releases their natural oils and enhances their flavors. Freshly ground spices offer a more robust and aromatic taste compared to pre-ground versions. Whether it's cumin, coriander, or peppercorns, using a pestle and mortar can elevate the flavor profile of your dishes. Plus, grinding your own spices allows you to create custom blends tailored to your taste preferences.

Flavor is the essence of memorable meals. By

incorporating these tips and experimenting with different combinations, you can create plant-based dishes that are not only nutritious but also bursting with taste. It's all about layering flavors and using quality ingredients to achieve the best results.

In this chapter, we equipped ourselves with a variety of tips and tricks to enhance our mood-food experience. Now, you're ready to apply these insights more specifically. The next chapter is dedicated to understanding how we can tailor our newfound knowledge to address particular mental health conditions.

Food & Mood

Depression

When feeling weighed down by symptoms of depression it can be difficult to find the energy to get out of bed, let alone try new strategies to improve our mood. But some hopeful new studies have demonstrated that small steps toward including healthy foods can help us feel happier. The Antidepressant Foods Study[22], in particular, investigates which foods are the most nutrient dense sources of nutrients that play a role in the prevention and recovery from depressive disorders. It provides a helpful list of "antidepressant plant foods."

Though there are a variety of factors that contribute to depressive states, new and exciting research is helping us further understand the connection between nutrition and depression. It is clear that nutrients—vitamins, minerals, amino acids, and omega-3 fatty acids—play a key role in how well our bodies produce the neurochemicals, like serotonin, that we need for a balanced mood. Due to the additional fiber and phytonutrients found in plants compared to supplements, it is best to try and get most of these nutrients from food as opposed to supplements.

---

[22] https://www.ncbi.nlm.nih.gov/pmc/articles/ PMC6147775/

Exercise, therapy, meditation, and socializing with supportive people in our lives can help improve our mood. Adding more plant-based foods, high in specific nutrients, to our diet is another tool we can use in the treatment of mood disorders.

Key Nutrients to Focus On:
Vitamins: B1, B2, B3, B6, B9, B12, A, and C
Minerals: Iron, magnesium, zinc, and selenium.

Top 10 Plant Foods for Depression
1. **Avocado**: Rich in healthy fats and B vitamins, which can help ward off depression by supporting the nervous system; the healthy fats also promote gut health.
2. **Leafy greens** (such as spinach, kale, Swiss chard, and turnip greens): Contain folic acid and other B vitamins which are vital for proper brain function and maintenance of mental health.
3. **Tomatoes**: Contain lycopene which helps guard against depression, as well as being a good source of vitamin C and potassium.
4. **Nuts and seeds** (such as walnuts, almonds, sunflower seeds): Abundant in Omega-3 fatty acids; these fatty acids support the nervous system and gut health, as well as the brain's ability to regulate mood.
5. **Blueberries**: Rich in antioxidants and vitamin C, which help protect against oxidative stress and reduce inflammation, playing a vital role in preserving mental health.
6. **Quinoa**: A complete protein source rich in

magnesium, zinc, B vitamins, and folate, important for energy and brain health

7. **Garlic**: Contains allicin, which helps reduce inflammation, a contributing factor for depression; also important to promote gut health.
8. **Sweet potatoes**: Provide our bodies with complex carbohydrates and fiber, contributing to balanced mood and energy, as well as being a source of vitamins A, C, and E.
9. **Mushrooms**: A natural source of Vitamin D, essential for boosting mood; they are also a great source of B vitamins, folate, selenium, and zinc, which all serve to aid mental health.
10. **Coconut oil**: A great source of healthy fats that nourish the brain and reduce inflammation; it can also aid in gut health.

Sample Plant-Based Menu for Depression

Breakfast: Tofu Scramble

Ingredients:
- 1/2 ripe avocado, sliced
- 1 cup fresh spinach (or a mix of kale and Swiss chard), roughly chopped
- 3 mushrooms
- 1/4 cup red bell pepper, chopped
- 2 tablespoon coconut oil (or olive oil)
- 1 block firm tofu, crumbled
- 1/2 onion, diced
- 1/2 teaspoon turmeric
- 1 tablespoon tamari/soy sauce (or 1 tsp black salt for more egg-like flavor)

- 1-2 tablespoon nutritional yeast
- 1 teaspoon garlic salt
- 1 teaspoon onion powder
- Pepper to taste

Instructions:
1. In a skillet, heat the oil over medium heat. Once hot, add the onion and sauté until fragrant.
2. Add the bell pepper and sauté for a few minutes.
3. Add the mushrooms and sauté for 2-3 minutes.
4. Add the crumbled tofu to the skillet. Add spices, soy sauce, and nutritional yeast and mix well. Sauté for about 3-4 minutes until the tofu is heated through.
5. Add the spinach to the skillet and sauté until wilted.
6. Add tomatoes to the skillet, stirring everything together. Season with pepper.
7. Top with avocado slices.

Lunch: Quinoa Stuffed Mushrooms

Ingredients:
- 8 large mushrooms (large chestnut or baby portobellos work well)
- 1 cup cooked quinoa
- 1/4 cup chopped almonds
- 1/4 cup chopped walnuts
- 1 tablespoon nutritional yeast
- 2 tablespoons coconut oil
- 1 garlic clove, minced
- Salt and pepper to taste

Instructions:
1. Preheat oven to 350F/180C.
2. Remove stems from mushrooms—set stems aside to use in stir-fry, soup, etc.
3. In a medium bowl, combine quinoa, almonds, walnuts, nutritional yeast, coconut oil, garlic, salt, and pepper. Mix until well combined.
4. Stuff each mushroom with the quinoa mixture and place on a baking sheet.
5. Bake for 25 minutes.

Dinner: Sweet Potato Black Bean Burrito

Ingredients:
- 1 medium sweet potato, diced
- 1/2 cup cooked black beans
- 1/2 cup dark leafy greens (kale, spinach, etc.), chopped
- 1/4 cup cooked quinoa
- 1/4 cup salsa
- 1/4 cup diced red onion
- 1 tablespoon coconut oil
- 1-2 whole wheat tortillas
- Salt and pepper to taste

Instructions:
1. Preheat oven to 425F/220C.
2. Toss sweet potatoes with melted coconut oil, salt, and pepper.
3. Place on baking sheet and bake for 20-30 minutes.
4. In a medium bowl, combine black beans, greens, quinoa, tomatoes, red onion, salsa. Mix

until well combined.

5.   Once sweet potatoes are finished, warm a tortilla, and fill with the bean mixture and sweet potatoes.

Incorporating a balanced diet rich in specific nutrients can be a powerful tool in targeting symptoms of depression. The growing evidence linking nutrition and mental well-being underscores the importance of our dietary choices. While therapy and meditation can be instrumental, the foods we consume, such as avocados, leafy greens, and nuts, offer foundational support.

Anxiety

Anxiety can both motivate and paralyze us. What we eat and drink can have an almost immediate effect on our levels of anxiety. Choosing plant-based foods rich in specific vitamins, eating lean proteins, and improving gut health can be instrumental in helping our body, brain, and nervous-system feel more relaxed.

While a variety of factors contribute to anxious states, new and exciting research is shedding light on the connection between nutrition and anxiety. Specifically, it's revealing the positive impact that fruits and vegetables have on decreasing symptoms.[23] It is clear that nutrients play a key role in how well our bodies produce the neurochemicals like GABA needed to help us feel calm. Additionally, recent insights highlight the importance of healthy fats (such as omega-3 fatty acids) and fermented foods (like plant-based yogurt and kimchi) in promoting a calm and stable state for both our gut and our nerves.

Exercise, therapy, breathing exercises, and meditation can help cultivate serenity in our daily lives. Adding more plant-based foods, high in specific nutrients, to

---

[23] https://www.ncbi.nlm.nih.gov/pmc/articles/
PMC8706568/

our diet is another tool we can use in the treatment of anxiety and stress-related disorders.

Key Nutrients to Focus On:
Vitamins: B1, B3, B5, B6, B9, A, C, D, and E
Minerals: Magnesium and selenium

Top 10 Plant Foods for Anxiety
1. **Avocado:** Packed with B vitamins, avocados are essential for the nerves and brain cells, which can be strained during times of anxiety. Its high content of omega-3 fatty acids can boost serotonin levels in the brain, a neurotransmitter responsible for mood regulation.
2. **Cauliflower**: As a rich source of B vitamins, cauliflower plays a key role in the synthesis of neurotransmitters that combat depression and anxiety. It also promotes overall brain health.
3. **Almonds**: With their high magnesium content, almonds can assist in regulating the nervous system, helping to alleviate symptoms of anxiety. Magnesium also promotes muscle relaxation which can be beneficial during tense moments.
4. **Blueberries**: These small berries are loaded with antioxidants and vitamin C, which have been shown to provide a defense against stress and anxiety-related free radicals. They also promote neuroprotective benefits.
5. **Sweet Potatoes**: Apart from their range of vitamins, the complex carbohydrates in sweet potatoes help increase the production of serotonin, a neurotransmitter that exerts a

calming effect.

6. **Plant-Based Yogurt**: The live cultures present in yogurts help maintain a balanced gut microbiome, which in turn plays a crucial role in the production of mood-regulating neurotransmitters like serotonin.

7. **Chia Seeds**: These tiny seeds are rich in omega-3 fatty acids, which have been linked to reduced inflammation and lower anxiety levels. They also support brain function and mood regulation.

8. **Spinach**: Packed with magnesium, spinach can help improve the body's response to stress and enhance sleep quality, which is crucial for managing anxiety. It also contains folate which contributes to neurotransmitter synthesis.

9. **Flax Seeds**: Another source of omega-3 fatty acids, flax seeds can assist in reducing inflammation, which is often elevated in those with anxiety. The magnesium in flax seeds also contributes to a calmer and clearer mind.

10. **Oats**: Known to be a great source of fiber, oats ensure a steady release of energy, preventing blood sugar spikes that can lead to anxiety. Their rich magnesium content supports nervous system function, further alleviating symptoms of stress and anxiety.

Sample Plant-Based Menu for Anxiety

Breakfast: Avocado Toast

Ingredients:
- 2 slices of whole grain bread

- 1 ripe avocado
- 1 teaspoon ground flaxseed
- Squeeze of lemon
- Handful of blueberries
- 1 teaspoon ground chia seeds
- Salt and pepper (optional)

Instructions:
1. Toast the slices of bread and set aside
2. Mash the avocado
3. Mix in flaxseed, chia seeds, and blueberries
4. Spread the mixture onto the toasted slices
5. Drizzle with lemon and season with salt and pepper (optional)

Lunch: Middle Eastern Chickpeas and Sweet Potatoes with Yogurt Dressing

Ingredients:
- 1 medium-sized sweet potato
- 1 cup of spinach
- 1 can (14 oz) of chickpeas, drained and rinsed
- 2 cloves of garlic, minced
- 2 tablespoons olive oil
- Salt and pepper to taste
- 1/2 cup plant-based yogurt
- 1 tablespoon tahini
- 1 tablespoon lemon juice
- 1/2 teaspoon ground cumin
- Optional: whole wheat pita bread
- *Optional*: fresh herbs such as parsley or mint for garnish
- *Optional:* a sprinkle of sumac or paprika for

added flavor
- Serve as a salad or in a pita pocket

Instructions:
1. Prepare the sweet potato: Dice the sweet potato into small cubes. In a large skillet, heat 1 tablespoon of olive oil over medium heat. Add the diced sweet potato and sauté for about 8-10 minutes or until they're almost cooked through and have a slight golden brown color. Remove them from the skillet and set them aside to cool.
2. Prepare the chickpeas: In the same skillet, add the remaining tablespoon of olive oil and minced garlic. Sauté for about 30 seconds until fragrant. Add the chickpeas, season with salt and pepper, and sauté for another 5-6 minutes until they're slightly crispy. Remove from heat and let them cool.
3. Prepare the dressing: In a small bowl, whisk together the plant-based yogurt, tahini, lemon juice, and ground cumin until smooth.
4. Assemble the salad: In a large mixing bowl, combine the cooled sweet potato, chickpeas, and fresh spinach. Drizzle the dressing over the top and gently toss to combine.
5. Garnish and serve: Transfer the salad to a serving dish. Garnish with fresh herbs and a sprinkle of sumac or paprika if desired. Serve immediately, or chill in the refrigerator for about 30 minutes before serving if preferred.

Dinner: Almond and Spinach Pesto Pasta with Roasted Cauliflower

Ingredients:
- 8 oz (about 2 cups) of your preferred pasta (whole wheat, gluten-free, etc.)
- 1 cup fresh spinach, packed
- 1/3 cup almonds, preferably roasted
- 2 cloves garlic
- 1/4 cup extra virgin olive oil
- 1 cup cauliflower florets
- Salt and pepper, to taste
- 1-2 tablespoons nutritional yeast
- 1 tablespoon lemon juice

Instructions:
1. Preheat your oven to 425°F (220°C).
2. In a bowl, toss the cauliflower florets with a tablespoon of olive oil, salt, and pepper. Spread them on a baking sheet and roast in the oven for 20 minutes or until golden and tender.
3. While the cauliflower is roasting, bring a large pot of salted water to boil. Add the pasta and cook according to the package instructions until al dente. Drain and set aside.
4. In a food processor or blender, combine the spinach, almonds, garlic, lemon juice, the remaining olive oil, and nutritional yeast (if using). Process until smooth. If the mixture is too thick, you can add a little more olive oil or water. Season with salt and pepper.
5. Toss the cooked pasta with the spinach and almond pesto. Gently fold in the roasted cauliflower and serve.

Incorporating these nutrient-rich foods into our daily

meals can be a step forward in managing anxiety. Coupled with other holistic approaches, a balanced diet can pave the way for a calmer, more centered life.

Libido

There is an interplay between our libido and many other mental health issues. Stress and anxiety, mood, lack of sleep, and mental tension can all have an impact on sexual desire and performance. If feeling low energy when it comes to bedroom activities, we might benefit from foods that help spice things up.

Though much of the current research on food and mood is focused on anxiety and depression, as the field of nutritional psychology expands we will likely see more studies that help us understand the link between diet, mental health, and sexual health. It is clear that nutrients—vitamins, minerals, amino acids, and omega 3 fatty acids—play a key role in how well our bodies produce sex hormones and neurochemicals necessary for mental wellness and physical stamina.

Sex therapy, meditation, tantra practices, and exercise can strengthen our libido and enhance our sex life. And though increasing the amount of plant-based food in our diet is sexy in itself, targeting specific nutrients may help us feel sexier, too.

Key Nutrients to Focus On:
Vitamins: B1, B3, B6, B9, and E
Minerals: Selenium, zinc, and magnesium

Top 10 Plant Foods for Libido

1. **Reishi Mushrooms**: Boosts circulation, hormonal balance, and energy levels.
2. **Maca Root**: A known aphrodisiac from Peru that improves sex drive.
3. **Nuts**: High in zinc and B vitamins, they regulate hormone levels.
4. **Bananas**: Source of vitamins B and C, important for improving sex drive.
5. **Flaxseeds**: High in zinc, they aid testosterone production.
6. **Avocados**: Contains healthy fats and vitamin E, boosting libido.
7. **Oats**: High in magnesium, they increase testosterone levels and help with erectile dysfunction.
8. **Asparagus**: Source of vitamins B and E, aiding overall sexual health.
9. **Beets**: High in nitrates, folate, magnesium, and vitamins B6 and C, they boost testosterone levels.
10. **Dark Chocolate**: Contains vitamins and minerals that aid in physical and mental arousal.

Sample Plant-Based Menu for Libido

Breakfast: Oat and Banana Porridge

Ingredients:
- 1 cup rolled oats
- 1 large ripe banana, mashed
- 2 cups plant-based milk (or half water, half PB milk)

- 1 tablespoon flaxseeds
- 1-2 tablespoons agave syrup or maple syrup (adjust to taste)
- 1/2 teaspoon ground cinnamon
- 1/4 cup of your favorite nuts, chopped
- Dark chocolate (optional)
- Plant-Based Yogurt (optional)

Instructions:
1. In a pot, bring the plant-based milk to a low boil.
2. Add oats, mashed banana, and flaxseeds, reducing the heat and letting it simmer for about 10 minutes or until oats are soft.
3. Stir in agave/syrup and chopped nuts
4. Sprinkle with cinnamon and top with grated chocolate and a dollop of yogurt (is using).

Lunch: Avocado Citrus Salad

Ingredients:
- 2 cups chopped romaine lettuce
- 1 orange, peeled and segmented
- 1 grapefruit, peeled and segmented
- 1 ripe avocado, sliced
- 1/2 teaspoon maca root powder
- 2 tablespoon olive oil
- Salt and pepper to taste

Instructions:
1. In a large salad bowl, combine lettuce, orange segments, grapefruit segments, and avocado slices.

2. Drizzle with olive oil and sprinkle with maca root powder.
3. Season with salt and pepper.
4. Gently toss the ingredients together and serve immediately.

Dinner: Warm Lentil Asparagus Salad

Ingredients:
- 1 cup cooked green, black, or brown lentils
- 2 tablespoons extra virgin olive oil
- 1/2 yellow onion, diced
- 1 large beet, chopped
- 1/2 bunch asparagus, chopped
- 4 medium carrots, chopped
- 1/2 bunch lacinato kale, ribs removed & chopped
- Handful of chopped parsley
- 1/2 cup plant-based cream
- Sea salt and black pepper to taste
- *Optional*: reishi mushrooms

Instructions:
1. In a large sauté pan, heat the olive oil over medium-high heat. Add the onion, beets, and carrots. Cook for about 10 minutes, stirring occasionally.
2. Add the asparagus to the pan and continue to cook for an additional 5 minutes.
3. Mix in the lentils and kale. Cook until the kale is wilted and the lentils are heated through, which should take about 2 minutes.
4. Season the mixture with salt and pepper to taste.

5. To serve, drizzle the plant-based cream on top and sprinkle with the chopped parsley.
6. Note: reishi mushrooms can be added for an extra libido boost. If using, add them along with the asparagus.

By focusing on these nutrient-rich foods, we can enhance our libido and overall well-being. A balanced diet, combined with other holistic practices, can lead to a more fulfilling and energetic intimate life.

Mental Fatigue

Often we rely on stimulants like coffee to power through the day and override brain fog. Yet, by inserting certain foods at the right time of day, we get more sustained mental clarity and focus, avoiding the crashes and the need for yet another round of Starbucks.

The effects of food on our mental processes are almost immediate. Overloading on carb-rich foods, especially during the first two meals of the day, can lead to brain fog. While carbs are essential for energy, we often neglect protein, a key macronutrient vital for the production of neurotransmitters like norepinephrine that aid mental stamina, concentration, and focus.

Many plant-based foods are rich in protein, including beets, avocado, onion, broccoli, asparagus, corn, and peas. Additionally, these foods contain micronutrients that support our bodies in producing the neurotransmitters essential for mental sharpness.

Key Nutrients to Focus On:
Vitamins: B1, B3, B5, B6, and B9
Minerals: Iron, magnesium, and zinc

Top 10 Plant Foods for Mental Clarity
1. **Beets**: Improve cognitive processes due to high

folate content and are a source of nitrates that enhance memory.

2. **Walnuts**: Contain antioxidants linked to improved cognitive function.
3. **Blueberries**: Rich in antioxidants and anthocyanins that boost brain function.
4. **Avocado**: Packed with healthy fats and fiber that fuel the brain.
5. **Hemp Seeds**: Contain essential fatty acids vital for optimal brain performance.
6. **Dark Chocolate**: Contains antioxidants and neurotransmitters that enhance brain function.
7. **Coconut Oil**: Features medium-chain triglycerides linked to improved mental clarity.
8. **Leafy Greens**: Rich in B-vitamins essential for proper brain function.
9. **Sunflower Seeds**: Contain vitamin E linked to improved cognitive performance.
10. **Chia Seeds**: A source of omega-3 fatty acids vital for brain health.

Sample Plant-Based Menu for Mental Clarity

Breakfast: Chocolate Avocado Smoothie

Ingredients:
- 1 cup plant-based milk
- 1 frozen banana
- 1/2 cup blueberries
- 1 tablespoon cocoa powder
- 1 cup spinach
- 1 tablespoon chia seeds
- 1/2 teaspoon cinnamon
- 1/4 cup walnuts

Instructions:
1. Place all ingredients in a blender.
2. Blend on high until smooth and creamy.
3. Pour into a glass and enjoy!

Lunch: Hemp and Avocado Salad

Ingredients:
- 1 cup cooked brown rice
- 1/4 cup almonds (tamari roasted work well!), roughly chopped
- 1 cup spinach, chopped
- 2 tablespoons hemp seeds
- 1 ripe avocado, diced
- 1 tablespoon lemon juice
- 1 tablespoon olive oil
- 2 teaspoons balsamic vinegar
- Salt and pepper, to taste

Instructions:
1. In a large bowl, combine brown rice, almonds, hemp seeds, and diced avocado.
2. In a small bowl, whisk together the lemon juice, olive oil, balsamic vinegar, salt, and black pepper.
3. Pour the dressing over the rice mixture and toss to combine well.

Dinner: Beet and Leafy Greens Stir-Fry with Sunflower Seeds

Ingredients:

- 2 tablespoons coconut oil
- 2 medium beets, diced
- 3 cups mixed leafy greens (like spinach, kale, or chard), roughly chopped
- 1/4 cup sunflower seeds
- 2 cloves garlic, minced
- 1/4 cup red onion, sliced
- 1 tablespoon tamari/soy sauce
- 1 tablespoon lemon juice
- Salt and pepper, to taste
- Grain of your choice (quinoa, millet, barley, farro, etc.), cooked

Instructions:

1. Heat coconut oil in a large skillet over medium heat.
2. Add the diced beets and cook for about 8-10 minutes, or until they start to soften.
3. Add the sliced red onion and minced garlic to the skillet, and sauté for another 2 minutes.
4. Stir in the leafy greens and cook until they're just wilted.
5. Drizzle the stir-fry with tamari, and lemon juice. Toss everything together.
6. Serve the stir-fry in bowls over cooked grains, topped with sunflower seeds. Season with salt and pepper as desired. Enjoy!

Incorporating these nutrient-rich foods into our daily meals can be a transformative step towards enhancing mental clarity and dispelling brain fog. By prioritizing a balanced intake of proteins, vitamins, and essential minerals, we not only nourish our bodies but also fortify our minds against the daily challenges. As we move away from quick fixes like caffeine and turn to nature's bounty, we pave the way for sustained focus and sharper cognition.

Sleep

Not getting enough rest can wreak havoc on daily life. But what if what we are eating during the day is contributing to those fitful nights of sleep? Adding certain foods that help with serotonin production (which converts to melatonin) can be a good place to start if we want to catch more Zzzs.

Often when we consider improving our sleep we target our pre-sleep routine: things like drawing the black-out curtains, turning down the room temperature, using blue light filters on our screens, and winding down with low-key activities like reading or meditation. However, a lot of these strategies may work even better if we are supporting our bodies with the right foods to help us get proper amounts of melatonin, the hormone that regulates our sleep-wake cycle.

There aren't a lot of foods that are directly related to melatonin production (though check out cherries below). But since "leftover" serotonin gets converted to melatonin at night, eating foods that support our serotonin system can be a great way to help our bodies better transition to sleep-mode at the end of the day. One way to do this is by mixing high-tryptophan foods with carbs. Foods high in protein, iron, B2, and B6 all tend to contain large amounts of tryptophan.

Key Nutrients to Focus On:
Vitamins: B2, B3, B6, B9, C, D, and E
Minerals: Magnesium, iron, and zinc

Top 10 Foods for Better Sleep
1. **Bananas**: Packed with potassium, magnesium, and tryptophan which can aid relaxation.
2. **Chickpeas**: A source of protein, fiber, iron, and magnesium, all essential for optimal relaxation.
3. **Almonds**: Contain nutrients like magnesium, calcium, potassium, and tryptophan known for promoting a calm mind.
4. **Cherries**: Rich in melatonin and antioxidants that aid in improving sleep quality.
5. **Oatmeal**: A prime source of complex carbohydrates and magnesium, which can help in soothing the nervous system.
6. **Turmeric**: Features curcumin which helps in regulating melatonin levels, essential for sleep.
7. **Sweet Potatoes**: Loaded with complex carbohydrates and magnesium, known for promoting relaxation.
8. **Green Leafy Vegetables**: Abundant in magnesium, potassium, and calcium, all of which are vital for a calm system.
9. **Lentils**: Rich in fiber, protein, and magnesium, which together can help in fostering relaxation.
10. **Herbal Teas**: Contains a mix of micronutrients and antioxidants known for their relaxing properties.

Sample Plant-Based Menu for Better Sleep

Breakfast: Oatmeal with Cherries and Almond Milk

Ingredients:
- 1 cup rolled oats
- 2 cups almond milk
- 1 cup fresh or frozen cherries, halved and pitted
- 1-2 tablespoons agave or maple syrup (adjust based on desired sweetness)
- 1 tablespoon chia seeds
- 1/4 cup chopped almonds
- Pinch of salt

Instructions:
1. In a saucepan, bring almond milk and a pinch of salt to a simmer over medium heat.
2. Add oats and cook for 5 minutes, stirring occasionally.
3. Add cherries, agave, chia seeds, and chopped almonds.
4. Cook for an additional 3-5 minutes or until the oats are tender and creamy. Serve warm.

Lunch: Chickpea and Greens Salad

Ingredients:
- 1 cup chickpeas (cooked or canned)
- 2 cups mixed greens (e.g., spinach, arugula, kale)
- 1 medium tomato, diced
- 1/2 cucumber, diced

- 1 bell pepper, diced
- 2 tablespoons olive oil
- 1 tablespoon balsamic vinegar
- 1/2 teaspoon turmeric
- 1 clove garlic, minced
- Salt and pepper, to taste

Instructions:
1. In a large bowl, combine chickpeas, greens, tomatoes, cucumbers, and bell peppers.
2. In a small bowl, whisk together olive oil, balsamic vinegar, minced garlic, turmeric, salt, and pepper.
3. Pour dressing over the salad and toss to combine.

Dinner: Sweet Potato and Lentil Curry

Ingredients:
- 2 tablespoons olive oil
- 2 cloves garlic, minced
- 1 medium onion, diced
- 1 teaspoon ground cumin
- 1 teaspoon ground coriander
- 1/2 teaspoon turmeric
- 1 cup cooked lentils
- 1 large sweet potato, diced
- 1 can (400ml) coconut milk
- 1-2 tablespoons tamari/soy sauce
- Pepper, to taste
- Brown rice, cooked
- *Optional*: fresh cilantro or parsley, chopped

Instructions:
1. Heat olive oil in a large skillet or saucepan over medium heat.
2. Sauté garlic and onion until translucent, about 3-4 minutes.
3. Add ground cumin, coriander, and turmeric; cook for another 1-2 minutes until fragrant.
4. Add the cooked lentils, diced sweet potato, soy sauce, and coconut milk to the pan.
5. Bring the mixture to a gentle simmer and let it cook for about 15-20 minutes or until the sweet potatoes are tender. Adjust seasoning with soy sacue and pepper.
6. Serve warm over rice, garnished with fresh herbs like cilantro or parsley if desired.

A holistic approach to sleep involves not just our nighttime routines but also the foods we consume throughout the day. By incorporating nutrient-rich, plant-based foods that support serotonin and melatonin production, we can naturally enhance our body's ability to transition into restful sleep. Coupled with other sleep-enhancing practices, a balanced diet can pave the way for rejuvenating nights and more energized days.

Having explored how to tailor our dietary choices to specific mental health conditions, we now venture into a broader, yet deeply interconnected realm. The upcoming chapter invites you to expand your perspective beyond personal well-being to embrace a more holistic approach. Here, we delve into how plant-based eating not only nurtures our own health but also contributes to a better world. We'll connect the dots between our individual choices and the larger tapestry of life, underscoring how our food decisions can be powerful acts of purpose and responsibility.

Bigger Picture

Meaning Making

We are all part of a complex, interdependent ecosystem, from the smallest microorganism to the largest mammal, from the tiniest seed to the tallest tree. And our choices, including what we eat, have far-reaching implications for this intricate web of life.

Choosing a plant-based diet is more than a personal health decision; it's a powerful choice that can contribute to a better world. And when we make choices that provide a sense of purpose or meaning we get an emotional boost. So, no matter what your diet preference, by focusing on including more plants and fewer animal products, you will be making an impact on the world as well as your mental health. Let's take a deeper look at how the meaningful choice to become more plant-based can benefit soil, planetary health, and offer compassionate care for other sentient beings.

First off, soil is not just dirt; it's a living, breathing entity teeming with billions of microorganisms that play a crucial role in our planet's health. Healthy soil is vital for growing nutritious food, storing carbon, and maintaining the planet's water cycle. However, conventional farming practices, particularly those associated with animal agriculture, often lead to soil degradation and loss of biodiversity. On the other hand, plant-based farming practices, such as crop rotation and organic farming, can help restore soil health, increase biodiversity, and sequester carbon, thereby mitigating climate change.

Next, let's consider the broader planetary health. The production of plant-based foods generally requires less land, water, and energy compared to animal-based foods. This means a lower carbon footprint and less strain on our planet's finite resources. Moreover, plant-based diets can help reduce deforestation and habitat loss, as less land is needed for growing crops to feed animals. By choosing a plant-based diet, we can contribute to a more sustainable and resilient food system that respects our planet's limits and ensures food security for future generations.

Finally, a plant-based diet contributes to compassionate care for other sentient beings. Animals are not mere commodities; they are sentient beings capable of feeling pain and experiencing emotions. By choosing a plant-based diet, we are choosing a path of compassion that respects all creatures' inherent worth and seeks to minimize harm and suffering. This compassionate choice extends beyond animals to include our fellow humans, as a plant-based diet can help address global issues such as hunger and malnutrition by making more efficient use of our planet's resources.

Adopting a plant-based diet is a powerful act of stewardship for our planet and its inhabitants. It's a meaningful choice that nourishes our body and spirit as we strive to live in harmony with the Earth and all its creatures. By choosing plant-based, we are choosing a healthier, more compassionate, and more sustainable world. And that's a choice worth making every single day.

Going Further

In the vast world of health and wellness, you've come to see how the gut is a central player in maintaining our overall well-being. While a plant-based diet is a powerful tool for gut health, it's just one piece of the puzzle. If you truly want to support your gut microbiome and, in turn, mental health, consider some of these options for extra credit:

Moderate Alcohol Consumption: Alcohol, in moderation, can have some health benefits. However, excessive drinking can disrupt the balance of bacteria in your gut, leading to issues like leaky gut syndrome and inflammation. As we've discussed, heavy alcohol consumption can also impair the absorption and metabolism of important B vitamins, such as thiamin and folate. These vitamins play an essential role in maintaining good mental health and cognitive function. If you drink, opt for a glass or two of red wine or beer, which contain polyphenols that can feed your gut bacteria.

Exercise: Physical activity is not only for the benefit of your muscles; it's for your microbes, too! Regular exercise can increase the diversity of your gut bacteria. A 2014 study published in the journal *Gut* found that athletes had a more diverse gut microbiome than non-athletes.[24] So, lace up those sneakers and get moving!

Meditation: The gut is often called the "second brain" due to its vast network of neurons. This means that our mental state can impact our gut health. Stress, for example, can disrupt gut bacteria and lead to digestive issues. Meditation, a practice that helps manage stress, can benefit gut health. A study published in the *General Psychiatry* journal earlier this year (2023) found that long-term meditation may be a factor in monks' gut microbiota being different from the control group.[25] According to the study, this microbial difference may be linked to lower risks of anxiety, depression, cardiovascular disease, and improved immune function.

Social Connection: Humans are social creatures, and our gut bacteria are no different. They thrive in diverse communities. Research has shown that social interactions can influence the composition of our gut microbiota. A 2014 study published in the journal *Nature* found that cohabitating partners had similar gut bacteria.[26] So, spending time with others might not just make you happier, it could make your gut healthier too.

Nature Exposure: Spending time in nature, whether walking in the park or hiking in the mountains, can benefit your gut health. The diverse array of microbes in natural environments can help diversify your own gut microbiota. Plus, the stress-

---

[24] https://gut.bmj.com/content/63/12/1913
[25] https://gpsych.bmj.com/content/36/1/e100893
[26] https://www.nature.com/articles/s41598-018-37298-9

reducing effects of nature can also benefit your gut.

Eat Dirt (Really!): This might sound strange, but hear me out. Our overly sanitized environments can limit our exposure to beneficial microbes. So, getting a little dirty can actually be good for your gut. This doesn't mean you should start eating handfuls of soil, but don't be afraid of a little dirt on your homegrown veggies. Consider leaving the skin on root vegetables like carrots and beets for the extra fiber, nutrients, and microbes.

Volunteering on Farms: This combines several of the above points - nature exposure, physical activity, and getting dirty. Plus, farms that use regenerative agricultural principles prioritize soil health, which means healthier and more diverse microbes to interact with. A 2020 study published in the journal *Science Daily* found that exposure to farm-like house dust protected against asthma by shaping the gut microbiota in early life.[27] Volunteering on a farm could be a win-win for you and your gut.

As you can see, gut health is a multifaceted issue that extends beyond diet alone. By incorporating these practices into your life, you can create a more holistic approach to health that benefits your gut and mind. Remember, every little bit helps, so don't feel like you need to do everything at once. Start with one or two changes and build from there. Your gut (and your brain) will thank you.

---

[27] https://www.sciencedaily.com/releases/2020/11/201102120033.htm

You're Worth It

You matter. Sounds trivial. It's not. You do. What happens in your body when you read this? Remember, whether you recoil or expand upon hearing these words, it is all information. No judgment. Let's go with the premise that this is true: YOU MATTER. If you tend to have an aversion to such a statement, you can still "act as if." Even if we struggle to see ourselves in the best light, we can perform actions and practice behaviors that support the idea that we matter. By doing so, we are informing ourselves of what is possible: we can care for ourselves simply because we deserve kindness, even if our belief system isn't on board with this notion.

Let's face it: ultimately, it is up to us; no one else is going to show up at the same level that we can for ourselves because others can't understand our unique situation as intimately as we do.

So, this becomes a fundamental aspect of change. We need to work toward believing that we are worth the effort. And I'm here to tell you: you are! So many possibilities get denied when we start from any other premise. Since change is difficult, let's do ourselves a favor and make room for the idea that by taking our own side, we create space for greater expansion—transformation toward the self we were created to be.

It's not easy.

Many people fall into the cycle of guilt and shame around how and what they eat. While diet and body image struggles are common, it is often a lonely experience. If you find yourself experiencing difficult emotions in response to your relationship with food, you are not alone.

One of the most important pieces to breaking the cycle of guilt and shame around eating is trying to accept and love ourselves exactly as we are. It is helpful to recognize that, although we may fall short of our diet goals and our bodies may change, our worth and value as human beings don't have to follow suit. We are much more than what our bodies look like. We are not flawed because we may have eaten too much seeking to block emotional pain. Seeking comfort when distressed is a normal human response. Learning to be compassionate to ourselves in times of struggle can go a long way toward self-acceptance.

Remember, change is hard and can be overwhelming. We may feel judged or scrutinized each time we attempt a new habit. But it's okay to struggle. The people offering their unsolicited critiques struggle, too. As much as possible, tune them out. Focus on what matters to you. Your path doesn't need to look like the next person's. We can practice self-care and self-compassion by celebrating anything that feels like progress to us. To be successful or acceptable, we don't have to fit Instagram's ideal of 'perfection.'

It can be helpful to focus on nourishment and satisfaction rather than guilt and shame. This means tuning into what makes us feel good—nutritionally, emotionally, and physically. To help with this, we can practice mindful eating—slowing down and being aware of what we eat and how it makes us feel.

Learning how to connect with our bodies and emotions is key to reducing stress and breaking the cycle. One method that can help is triggering the dopaminergic pathway. This pathway in the brain releases the neurotransmitter dopamine, which affects our pleasure reward center. When activated, dopamine helps us find the activity rewarding and pleasurable, leading us away from the emotional urge to eat.

For many people, emotional eating is a way of silencing the anxiety and negative emotions that overwhelm us. Here are some ways of triggering the dopaminergic pathway and helping us to break free of the cycle:

Exercise: Exercising releases endorphins into our bodies, which affects the dopaminergic pathway and helps to reduce stress. Regular exercise also helps reduce cortisol, the hormone that promotes food cravings.

Change Your Eating Habits: Emotional eating is often caused by unhealthy and irregular eating habits. By creating a consistent eating schedule and having healthy, balanced meals, we can reduce stress and make it easier to find healthy alternatives to emotional eating.

Engage in a Hobby: Pursuing a favorite hobby is a great way to trigger your dopaminergic pathway. Look for activities you enjoy, and set aside time to do things you love.

Practice Mindfulness: Mindfulness involves becoming aware of your thoughts, feelings, emotions, and sensations without judgment. It helps to reduce stress and improve focus. When done regularly, mindfulness can trigger your dopaminergic pathway and help us choose more productive activities over emotional eating.

Breaking the cycle of guilt and shame around eating can be a complex process. It takes time, patience, and self-compassion. It is important to find positive outlets that bring joy and engage in self-care activities that give us a greater sense of peace. Remember, you are more than just a body. You deserve love and acceptance no matter what.

Conclusion

An Ending, A Beginning

Through understanding the relationship between food and mood, it becomes evident that the choices we make at the dining table reverberate far beyond mere sustenance. Embracing a plant-based diet is more than just trying a new fad diet; it's a commitment to enhancing our mind, body, and spirit. Throughout our exploration, we've seen how our gut health, the foods we consume, and our emotions are deeply interconnected. The choices we make daily have the power to heal, rejuvenate, and uplift.

As we end here, and you continue on your plant-based path, here are a few actionable steps to guide your journey:

Mindful Eating: Dedicate one meal a day to savoring each bite. Be present and appreciate the nourishment it provides.

Education: Stay informed about the benefits of a plant-based diet. Knowledge empowers us to make better choices. I'll be sharing regular updates on my own discoveries over at healthymoods.org. Follow along so we can continue to learn together.

Experiment: Introduce one new plant-based dish into your diet every week. Variety keeps our meals exciting and nutritionally diverse.

Share: Discuss your journey with friends and family. Sharing your experiences can inspire others and provide you with a supportive community.

Thank you for joining me in this exploration. Your dedication to understanding the connection between diet and mental well-being is a testament to your commitment to a healthier, happier life. As you close this book, I hope the information stays with you, offering supportive guidance in your food choices. Remember, every bite offers the potential to nourish both body and mind.

Thank you for reading.

Health to your navel, marrow to your bones, peace and joy to your heart and brain!

Milton Keynes UK
Ingram Content Group UK Ltd.
UKHW030013010324
438562UK00014B/479